LOW - CARB RECIPES COOKBOOK

Delicious and Healthy Meals for Weight Loss and Vitality

By

Hubert April

Table of Content

Introduction

Welcome to **Low-Carbs Recipes Cookbook: Delicious and Healthy Meals for Weight Loss and Vitality**. This book is designed to be your ultimate guide to embracing a low-carb lifestyle without sacrificing taste or satisfaction. Whether you're new to low-carb eating or a seasoned pro, this collection of recipes will inspire you to enjoy wholesome, nutritious, and incredibly delicious meals every day.

In recent years, the benefits of a low-carb diet have become widely recognized and embraced by health enthusiasts and professionals alike. From aiding in weight loss and enhancing mental clarity to reducing inflammation and stabilizing blood sugar levels, cutting back on carbohydrates can lead to a healthier, more energetic life. However, the challenge often lies in finding recipes that are both low in carbs and rich in flavor. That's where this cookbook comes in, offering a wealth of options that make low-carb eating not just viable but delightful.

This cookbook is curated with a variety of recipes that cater to different tastes and preferences, ensuring that you'll find something delightful for every meal. From hearty breakfasts and satisfying lunches to savory dinners and indulgent desserts, each recipe is designed to be low in carbohydrates while rich in nutrients and flavors. We believe that food should be enjoyable, and eating healthy shouldn't mean compromising on taste.

Our goal is to make low-carb cooking accessible and enjoyable for everyone. You'll find easy-to-follow instructions, readily available ingredients, and practical tips to help you succeed in the kitchen. We've also included nutritional information for each recipe, so you can make informed choices that align with your dietary goals. Whether you're cooking for yourself, your family, or guests, these recipes are designed to impress and nourish.

In the opening chapters, you'll find essential information on understanding carbohydrates, the benefits of reducing them, and tips for stocking a low-carb pantry. We've also included practical advice on meal planning and preparation, so you can streamline your cooking process and make the most out of your ingredients.

As you delve into the recipes, you'll discover a world of flavors and textures that make low-carb eating a joy rather than a chore. Start your day with energizing breakfasts like Almond Flour Pancakes with Berries or Avocado and Bacon Egg Muffins. For lunch, enjoy light and lovely dishes like Zucchini Noodles with Pesto and Cherry Tomatoes or a refreshing Grilled Chicken and Avocado Salad. Dinner options include hearty and satisfying meals like Garlic Butter Shrimp with Zoodles and Baked Lemon Herb Salmon. And don't forget to treat yourself with decadent desserts like Chocolate Avocado Mousse and Coconut Flour Brownies.

We've also dedicated chapters to snacks, sauces, and drinks, ensuring that you have a comprehensive resource for every culinary need. From Spicy Roasted Chickpeas to Green Detox Smoothies, these recipes are perfect for keeping your energy levels up throughout the day.

To help you stay on track, we've included a 7-day meal plan and shopping list, making it easy to plan your week and stay committed to your low-carb lifestyle. You'll also find tips for eating out and making low-carb choices when dining away from home.

Embark on this culinary journey and discover how delicious low-carb living can be. Whether your goal is to lose weight, improve your health, or simply try something new, **Low-Carbs Recipes Cookbook** is here to support and inspire you every step of the way. Enjoy the journey to a healthier, happier you with these delicious and healthy meals designed for weight loss and vitality.

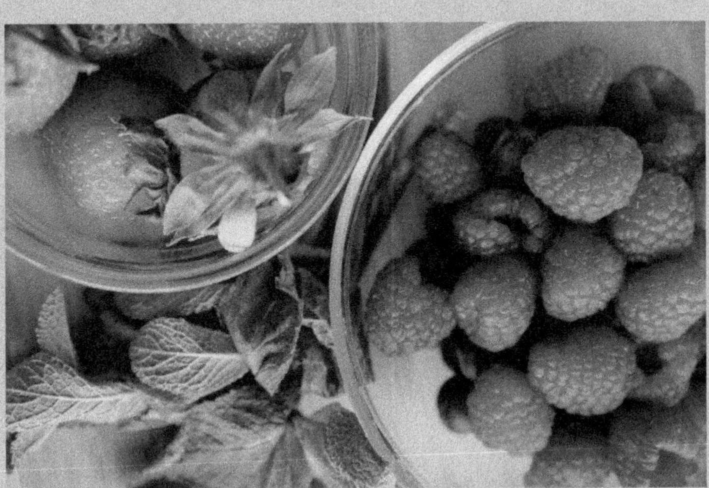

Getting Started

Understanding Carbohydrates

Carbohydrates are one of the three macronutrients essential to our diet, alongside proteins and fats. They are the body's primary source of energy, found in foods like grains, fruits, vegetables, and dairy products. However, not all carbohydrates are created equal. They fall into two general categories: simple and complex carbohydrates.

Simple carbohydrates are sugars that the body absorbs fast, causing blood sugar levels to increase dramatically. Common sources include:

- Candy and sweets
- Soda and sugary drinks
- Baked goods made with white flour, such as cakes, cookies, and pastries
- Ice cream and other sugary desserts

Complex Carbohydrates:

These are starches and fibers that take longer to digest, providing a more sustained energy release. They are found in:

- Whole grains such as oats, quinoa, and brown rice
- Legumes like black beans, chickpeas, and lentils
- Vegetables such as carrots, butternut squash, and sweet potatoes

In a low-carb diet, the focus is on reducing the intake of simple carbs and selecting complex carbs with a low glycemic index, which have a minimal impact on blood sugar levels. This approach helps in managing weight, reducing the risk of chronic diseases, and promoting overall health.

Benefits of a Low-Carb Diet

Adopting a low-carb lifestyle offers numerous health benefits:

1. **Weight Loss:** Weight reduction: Cutting back on carbohydrates causes the body to begin burning fat reserves for energy, which results in weight reduction. This process, known as ketosis, is a hallmark of many low-carb diets. Examples of successful low-carb diets include the ketogenic diet and the Atkins diet.

2. **Improved Blood Sugar Control:** A low-carb diet can stabilize blood sugar levels, making it beneficial for individuals with diabetes or insulin resistance. For instance, replacing white bread with leafy greens for sandwiches can significantly reduce carbohydrate intake.

3. **Enhanced Mental Clarity:** Many people report better focus and mental clarity when they reduce their carb intake. Foods like nuts, seeds,

and avocados provide healthy fats that support brain health.

4. **Reduced Inflammation:** A low-carb diet can help reduce inflammation in the body, lowering the risk of chronic diseases like heart disease and arthritis. Incorporating anti-inflammatory foods such as fatty fish, olive oil, and leafy greens can further enhance these benefits.

5. **Increased Energy Levels:** By avoiding the spikes and crashes associated with high-carb meals, many people experience more consistent energy levels throughout the day. Low-carb snacks like cheese sticks, hard-boiled eggs, and raw vegetables with hummus can help maintain steady energy.

Essential Low-Carb Ingredients

Stocking your kitchen with the right ingredients is crucial for success on a low-carb diet. The following are necessities to have on hand:

Proteins:

- Chicken breast and thighs
- Beef cuts like sirloin, ribeye, and ground beef
- Pork chops and tenderloin
- Fish such as salmon, tilapia, and sardines
- Eggs, tofu, and tempeh

Healthy Fats:

- Avocado and avocado oil
- Olive oil and coconut oil
- Nuts (almonds, walnuts, pecans) and seeds (chia, flax, sunflower)
- Nut butters, such as peanut and almond butters

Low-Carb Vegetables:

- leafy greens, such as Swiss chard, kale, and spinach
- Cruciferous vegetables such as broccoli, cauliflower, and Brussels sprouts
- Zucchini, bell peppers, mushrooms, and asparagus

Dairy and Alternatives:

- Cheese varieties (cheddar, mozzarella, goat cheese)
- Greek yogurt (unsweetened)
- Almond milk and coconut milk (unsweetened)

Pantry Staples:

- Almond flour, coconut flour, and flaxseed meal
- Chia seeds and hemp hearts
- Low-carb sweeteners, such as monk fruit, erythritol, and stevia

Herbs and Spices:

- Fresh and dried herbs: basil, oregano, thyme, rosemary
- Spices: cumin, paprika, turmeric, cinnamon, ginger

Tips for Stocking Your Low-Carb Pantry

A well-stocked pantry makes it easier to prepare low-carb meals without stress. Here are some tips:

1. **Organize by Category:** Group similar items together, such as oils, spices, and baking ingredients, to make them easy to find. To keep everything accessible and visible, use clear containers.
2. **Buy in Bulk:** Purchase non-perishable items like nuts, seeds, and flours in bulk to save money and ensure you always have them on hand. Consider joining a wholesale club for better deals.
3. **Label Everything:** Use clear labels on containers to quickly identify ingredients and their carb content. This helps in making quick decisions while cooking.
4. **Plan Ahead:** Keep a list of low-carb staples and check your inventory regularly to avoid running out of key ingredients. Update your shopping list as soon as you notice items running low.

Meal Planning and Preparation

Maintaining a low-carb diet requires careful meal planning and preparation.

1. **Make a Weekly Meal Plan**: Set aside time to organize your meals and snacks.
2. Choose recipes that you enjoy and fit your schedule. For example, if you know you have busy mornings, plan for quick breakfasts like chia seed pudding or egg muffins.
3. **Make a Shopping List**: Based on your meal plan, create a detailed shopping list to ensure you buy only what you need. Group items by category to make your shopping trip more efficient.
4. **Prep in Advance:** Prepare ingredients in advance, such as chopping vegetables, marinating meats, or cooking grains. This saves time and makes it easier to assemble meals during the week. For instance, batch-cook cauliflower rice and store it in the fridge for quick meals.
5. **Batch Cooking:** Cook large batches of meals and store them in portioned containers for easy access throughout the week. Consider making a big pot of soup or stew that you can enjoy for several days.
6. **Stay Flexible:** Be open to adjusting your meal plan based on what's available or in season. Flexibility helps you stay on track without feeling

restricted. If avocados are on sale, incorporate them into several meals that week.

By understanding carbohydrates, recognizing the benefits of a low-carb diet, and equipping yourself with the right ingredients and planning strategies, you'll be well on your way to a successful and enjoyable low-carb lifestyle. This foundation sets the stage for the delicious and nutritious recipes that follow in this cookbook.

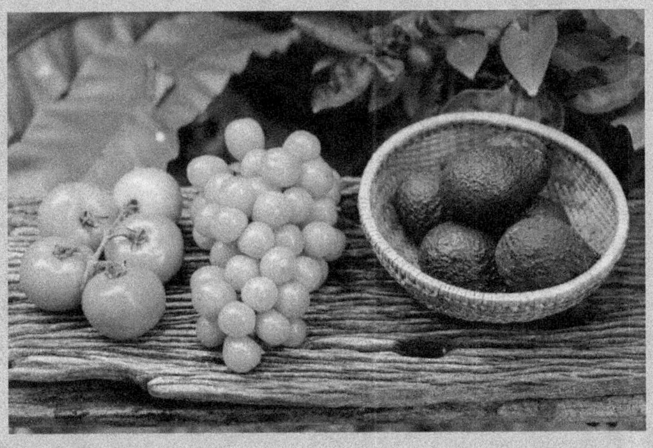

Breakfast Boosters

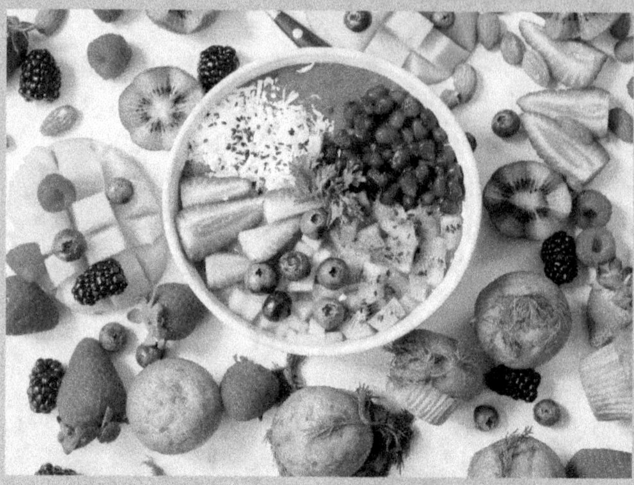

Breakfast is frequently considered the most important mess of the day, setting the tone for your energy situations and metabolism. In a low- carb diet, it's essential to start your day with refection's that aren't only low in carbohydrates but also rich in protein, healthy fats, and essential nutrients.

This chapter is devoted to furnishing you with a variety of succulent and nutritional breakfast options that will keep you satisfied and reenergized throughout the morning.

Classic Scrambled Eggs with Spinach and Feta

Scrambled eggs are a breakfast feta, and adding spinach and feta elevates this simple dish into a nutritional hustler.

Ingredients

- 3 large eggs
- 1 mug fresh spinach
- diced **soup spoons** atrophied feta rubbish
- 1 teaspoon of butter or olive oil
- Salt and pepper to taste

Instructions

- In a bowl, whisk the eggs until well combined. Season with salt and pepper.
- Toast the butter or olive oil in a skillet over medium heat.
- Add the spinach to the skillet and sauté until wilted.
- Pour the eggs into the skillet and cook, stirring gently, until the eggs are set but still soft.
- Sprinkle the feta cheese over the eggs and stir to combine. Serve incontinently.

Almond Flour Pancakes with Berries

These ethereal almond flour pancakes are a succulent low- carb volition to traditional pancakes, perfect for a weekend breakfast treat.

Ingredients

- 1 mug almond flour
- 2 large eggs
- ¼ mug unsweetened almond milk
- 1 tablespoon vanilla excerpt
- ½ tablespoon baking powder
- Pinch of salt
- Fresh berries and sugar-free syrup for serving

Instructions

In a mixing bowl combine the almond flour, baking powder, and salt.

In another bowl, whisk together the eggs, almond milk, and vanilla extract.

Pour the wet ingredients into the dry ingredients and stir until well combined.

Toast a non-stick skillet over medium heat and smoothly grease with butter or oil.

Pour ¼ mug of batter onto the skillet for each pancake. Cook until bubbles form on the face, also flip and cook until golden brown.

Serve the pancakes with fresh berries and a drizzle of sugar-free syrup.

Avocado and Bacon Egg Muffins

These savory egg muffins are perfect for meal fix, offering a quick and easy breakfast option that's packed with flavor and nutrients.

Ingredient

- 6 large eggs
- 1 ripe avocado
- 4 slices cooked bacon, crumbled
- ¼ mug shredded cheddar cheese
- Salt and pepper to taste
- cuisine spray

Instructions

- Preheat your Oven to 350 °F (175 °C). Spray a muffin tin with cuisine spray.
- In a large bowl, whisk the eggs and season with salt and pepper.
- Divide the avocado, bacon, and cheese evenly among the muffin mugs.
- Pour the beaten eggs into each muffin mug, filling about ¾ full.
- Bake for 20- 25 minutes, or until the eggs are set and the covers are golden.
- Allow the muffins to cool slightly before removing it, Store in the refrigerator for over to a week.

Chia Seed Pudding with Coconut Milk

This delicate and succulent chia seed pudding is a perfect make- ahead breakfast, offering a nutritional launch to your day.

Ingredients

- ¼ mug chia seeds
- 1 mug unsweetened coconut milk
- 1 tablespoon vanilla extract
- 1 teaspoon sugar-free sweetener (voluntary)
- Fresh berries or nuts for beating

Instructions

- In a bowl, combine the chia seeds, coconut milk, vanilla extract, and sweetener (if using).
- Stir well to combine, making sure the chia seeds are unevenly distributed.
- Cover the bowl and chill for at least 4 hours, or overnight, until the admixture has thickened.
- Stir the pudding before serving and top with fresh berries or nuts.

Low- Carb Smoothie Bowls

Smoothie bowls are a protean and succulent way to enjoy a nutrient- packed breakfast. Customize with your favorite low-carb condiments.

Ingredients

- ½ mug of unsweetened almond milk
- ½ avocado
- ½ mug firmed berries (similar as raspberries or strawberries)
- 1 scoop protein powder (voluntary)
- Sprinkle of spinach or kale

Topping Ideas

- Sliced almonds
- Unsweetened tattered coconut
- Chia seeds
- Fresh berries
- Sliced avocado

Instructions

- In a blender, combine the almond milk, avocado, firmed berries, protein powder, and greens. Mix until smooth.
- Pour the smoothie into a bowl.
- Add your favorite low- carb condiments and enjoy incontinently.

Savory Breakfast Bowls

A hearty and savory option for breakfast, these bowls can be customized with your favorite low- carb ingredients.

Ingredients

- 1 mug cooked cauliflower rice
- 2 large eggs
- ½ avocado, sliced
- ¼ mug salsa
- 2 soupspoons tattered cheese
- Fresh cilantro, diced
- Salt and pepper to taste

Instructions

- Toast the cauliflower rice in a skillet over medium heat until warmed through. Season with salt and pepper.
- In a separate skillet, cook the eggs to your choice (scramble, fried, or coddled).
- Assemble the bowl by placing the cauliflower rice at the bottom. Top with the eggs, avocado slices, salsa, and tattered cheese.
- Garnish with fresh cilantro and add more salt and pepper if desired.

Greek Yogurt with Nuts and Seeds

A simple yet satisfying breakfast, Greek yogurt outgunned with a variety of nuts and seeds provides a perfect balance of protein and healthy fats.

Ingredients

- 1 mug plain Greek yogurt
- 1 teaspoon chia seeds
- 1 teaspoon flaxseeds
- ¼ mug mixed nuts (almonds, walnuts, pecans)

- 1 tablespoon cinnamon
- 1 teaspoon sugar-free sweetener (voluntary)

Instructions:

- In a bowl, combine the Greek yogurt with chia seeds, flaxseeds, and mixed nuts.

- Sprinkle with cinnamon and sweetener if using.
- Stir well and enjoy immediately, or refrigerate for later.

Omelette with Mushrooms, Tomatoes, and Cheese

Omelettes are a versatile breakfast option, allowing you to incorporate a variety of low - carb vegetables and proteins.

Ingredients:

- 3 large eggs
- 1/4 cup mushrooms, sliced
- 1/4 cup cherry tomatoes, halved
- 1/4 cup shredded cheese (cheddar, mozzarella, or your choice)
- 1 tablespoon butter or olive oil
- Salt and pepper to taste

Instructions:

- In a bowl, whisk the eggs until well combined. Season with salt and pepper.
- Heat the butter or olive oil in a skillet over medium heat.

- Add the mushrooms and tomatoes to the skillet and sauté until softened.
- Pour the eggs into the skillet, tilting to spread evenly.
- Sprinkle the cheese over one half of the omelette.
- Cook until the eggs are set, then fold the omelette in half. Serve immediately.

Cottage Cheese with Fresh Herbs

Cottage cheese is a high-protein, low-carb option that can be enhanced with fresh herbs for added flavor.

Ingredients:

- 1 cup cottage cheese
- 1 tablespoon fresh parsley, chopped
- 1 tablespoon fresh dill, chopped
- 1 teaspoon lemon zest
- Salt and pepper to taste

Instructions

- In a bowl, combine the cottage cheese with parsley, dill, and lemon zest.
- Season with salt and pepper to taste.
- Stir well and enjoy immediately, or refrigerate for later.

These breakfast recipes are designed to provide a variety of options that are easy to prepare, delicious, and packed with the nutrients needed to start your day on the right foot. By incorporating these low-carb breakfasts into your routine, you'll be well-equipped to maintain your energy levels and stay on track with your dietary goals.

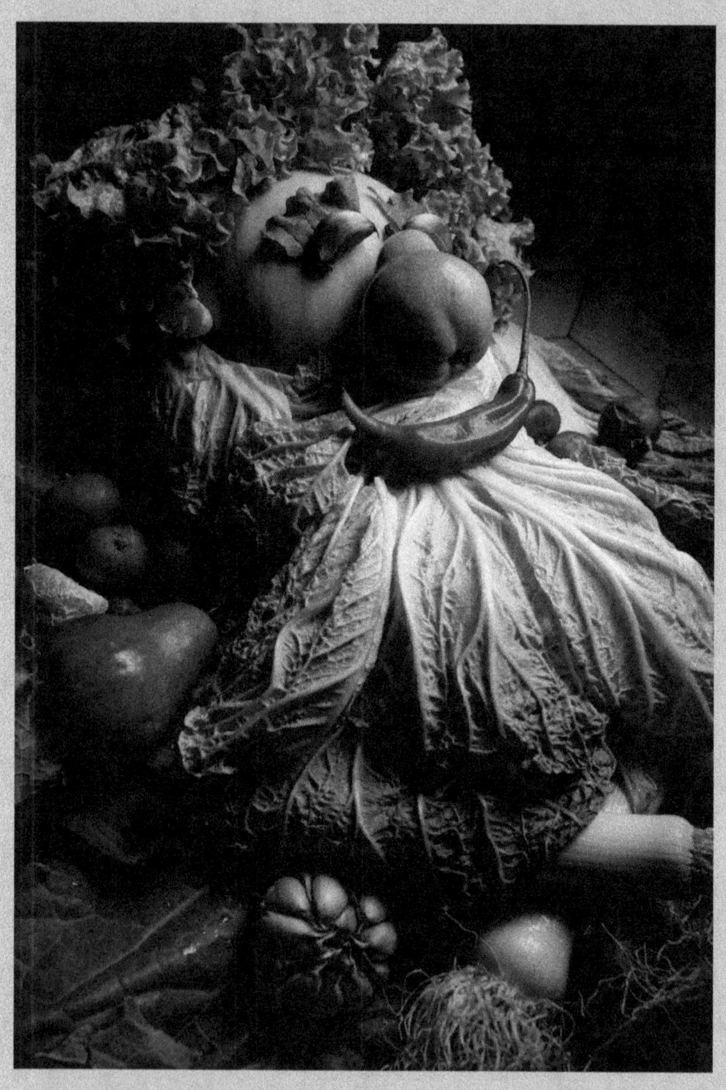

Light and Lovely Lunches

Lunch provides an excellent occasion to refuel your body with nutritional and satisfying meals. In this chapter, we present a variety of light and lovely lunch recipes that aren't only low in carbohydrates but also rich in protein, healthy fats, and fresh vegetables. These fashions are designed to keep you reenergized and satisfied throughout the noon, without the promptness that can come from high- carb meals.

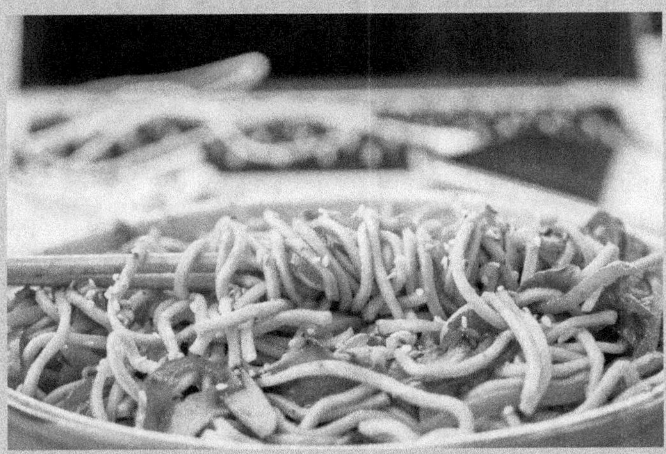

Zucchini Noodles with Pesto and Cherry Tomatoes

Zucchini noodles, also known as zoodles, are a fantastic low- carb option to traditional pasta. This dish combines the fresh flavors of homemade pesto with sweet cherry tomatoes for a stimulating and satisfying meal.

Ingredient

- 2 medium zucchinis, spiralized
- 1 mug cherry tomatoes, halved
- ½ mug of homemade or store-bought pesto
- ¼ mug grated Parmesan cheese
- 1 teaspoon olive oil
- Salt and pepper to taste

Instructions

- Toast the olive oil in a large skillet over medium heat.
- Add the zucchini noodles and cook for 2- 3 minutes until they're just tender.
- Add the cherry tomatoes and cook for another 1- 2 minutes.
- Remove from heat and toss the zoodles and tomatoes with pesto.
- Season with salt and pepper, and sprinkle with grated Parmesan cheese before serving.

Grilled Chicken and Avocado Salad

This grilled chicken and avocado salad is a hearty and nutritional option that's perfect for lunch. The delicate avocado pairs wonderfully with the grilled chicken and crisp vegetables.

Ingredients

- 2 boneless, skinless chicken breast
- 1 teaspoon olive oil
- 1 tablespoon garlic powder
- Salt and pepper to taste
- 4 mugs mixed green (spinach, arugula, and romaine)
- 1 avocado, sliced
- ½ mug cherry tomatoes, halved
- ¼ mug red onion, thinly sliced
- ¼ mug feta cheese, crumbled

Dressing

- ¼ mug olive oil
- 2 soupspoons balsamic vinegar
- 1 tablespoon Dijon mustard
- 1 garlic clove, diced
- Salt and pepper to taste

Instructions

- Preheat a grill or grill pan over medium-high heat.
- Season the chicken breasts with olive oil, garlic powder, salt, and pepper.
- Grill the chicken for 6- 7 minutes per side, or until completely cooked. Let it rest before slicing.
- In a large bowl, combine the mixed greens, avocado, cherry tomatoes, red onion, and feta cheese.

- In a small bowl, whisk together the dressing ingredients.
- Add the sliced chicken to the salad and drizzle with the dressing. Toss to combine and serve incontinently.

Cauliflower Fried Rice

Cauliflower fried rice is a low-carb option to traditional fried rice, packed with vegetables and flavor. This dish is quick to prepare and perfect for a satisfying lunch.

Ingredients

- 1 medium head of cauliflower, grated into rice-sized pieces
- 2 soupspoons sesame oil
- 1 small onion, minced
- 2 garlic cloves, diced
- 1 mug mixed vegetables (peas, carrots, bell peppers)
- 2 large eggs, beaten
- 2 soup spoons of soy sauce or tamari
- 1 teaspoon green onions, diced (voluntary)
- Salt and pepper to taste

Instructions

- Toast the sesame oil in a large skillet or wok over medium-high heat.
- Add the onion and garlic, and sauté until fragrant.
- Add the mixed vegetables and cook until tender.

- Push the vegetables to one side of the skillet and pour the beaten eggs into the other side. Scramble the eggs until cooked.
- Add the cauliflower rice to the skillet and stir to combine with the vegetables and eggs.
- Pour in the soy sauce and cook for another 3- 5 minutes until the cauliflower is tender.
- Season with salt and pepper, and garnish with green onions before serving.

Turkey and Cheese Lettuce Wraps

Lettuce wraps are a great way to enjoy the flavors of a sandwich without the carbs from bread. These Turkey and cheese wraps are quick to prepare and perfect for a light lunch.

Ingredients

- 8 large lettuce leaves (Romaine or iceberg)
- 8 slices turkey breast
- 4 slices cheese (cheddar, Swiss, or your choice)
- 1 avocado, sliced
- 1 small tomato, sliced
- ¼ mug mayonnaise or mustard
- Salt and pepper to taste

Instructions

- Lay the lettuce leaves flat on a clean surface.
- Spread a thin layer of mayonnaise or mustard on each leaf.

- Place a slice of turkey, cheese, avocado, and tomato on each leaf.
- Season with salt and pepper.
- Roll up the lettuce leaves, and put them away on the sides as you go, to form wraps.
- Secure with toothpicks if demanded, and serve incontinently.

Shrimp and Avocado Salad

This shrimp and avocado salad is light, stimulating, and packed with protein and healthy fats. It's perfect for a quick and satisfying lunch.

Ingredients

- 1 lb cooked shrimp, peeled and deveined
- 1 avocado, minced
- 1 cucumber, minced
- ½ red onion, thinly sliced
- ¼ mug cilantro, diced
- 1 soupspoons olive oil
- 1 teaspoon lime juice
- Salt and pepper to taste

Instructions

- In a large bowl, combine the shrimp, avocado, cucumber, red onion, and cilantro.
- In a small bowl, whisk together the olive oil and lime juice.
- Pour the dressing over the salad and toss to combine.

- Season with salt and pepper to taste. Serve incontinently.

Eggplant Roll-Ups with Ricotta and Spinach

These eggplant roll-ups are a succulent and low-carb option that's perfect for lunch. The combination of ricotta and spinach makes for a delicate and flavorful filling

Ingredients

- 2 medium eggplants, thinly sliced lengthwise
- 1 mug ricotta cheese
- 1 mug fresh spinach, diced
- 1 mug grated Parmesan cheese
- 1 egg, beaten
- 1 mug marinara sauce
- 1 teaspoon olive oil
- Salt and pepper to taste

Instructions

- Preheat your roaster to 375 °F (190 °C).
- Brush the eggplant slices with olive oil and season with salt and pepper.
- Grill the eggplant slices until tender, about 3- 4 minutes per side.
- In a bowl, combine the ricotta cheese, spinach, Parmesan cheese, and beaten egg.
- Season with salt and pepper.
- Spread a thin layer of the ricotta admixture onto each eggplant slice and roll up.

- Spread a thin layer of marinara sauce on the bottom of a baking dish.
- Place the eggplant roll-up seam-side down in the baking dish. Top with remaining marinara sauce.
- Bake for 20- 25 minutes until heated **through and the** cheese is bubbly and Serve.

Tuna Stuffed Avocados

Tuna stuffed avocados are a simple yet flavorful lunch option that's packed with protein and healthy fats.

Ingredients:

- 2 ripe avocados, halved and pitted
- 1 can tuna, drained
- 1/4 cup mayonnaise
- 1 tablespoon lemon juice
- 1 celery stalk, finely chopped
- 1/4 red onion, finely chopped
- Salt and pepper to taste

Instructions:

- In a bowl, combine the tuna, mayonnaise, lemon juice, celery, and red onion.
- Season with salt and pepper to taste.
- Spoon the tuna mixture into the avocado halves.
- Serve immediately, or chill for later.

Caprese Salad with Balsamic Glaze

This classic Italian salad is simple, fresh, and perfect for a light lunch. The combination of tomatoes, mozzarella, and basil is always a winner.

Ingredients:

- 4 ripe tomatoes, sliced
- 8 ounces fresh mozzarella, sliced
- Fresh basil leaves
- 2 tablespoons olive oil
- 1/4 cup balsamic vinegar
- Salt and pepper to taste

Instructions:

- Arrange the tomato and mozzarella slices on a platter, alternating between the two.
- Tuck basil leaves in between the slices.
- Drizzle with olive oil.
- In a small saucepan, heat the balsamic vinegar over medium heat until it reduces by half and becomes a glaze.
- Drizzle the balsamic glaze over the salad.
- Season with salt and pepper to taste. Serve immediately.

Chicken Caesar Salad

A classic Caesar salad made with grilled chicken breast is a hearty and satisfying lunch option. This version skips the croutons to keep it low-carb.

Ingredients:

- 2 boneless, skinless chicken breasts
- 1 tablespoon olive oil
- Salt and pepper to taste
- 6 cups Romaine lettuce, chopped
- 1/4 cup grated Parmesan cheese
- Caesar dressing (store-bought or homemade)
- Optional: 1 hard-boiled egg, sliced

Instructions:

- Preheat a grill or grill pan over medium-high heat.
- Season the chicken breasts with olive oil, salt, and pepper.
- Grill the chicken for 6-7 minutes per side, or until fully cooked. Let it rest before slicing.
- In a large bowl, combine the Romaine lettuce and Parmesan cheese.
- Add the sliced chicken and toss with Caesar dressing.
- Top with slices of hard-boiled egg if desired. Serve immediately.

These lunch recipes are designed to provide a variety of options that are easy to prepare, delicious, and packed with the nutrients needed to keep you energized and satisfied throughout the day. By incorporating these low-carb lunches into your routine, you'll be well-equipped to maintain your energy levels and stay on track with your dietary goals.

Delicious Dinners

Dinner is the perfect time to unwind and enjoy a satisfying meal that nourishes your body and delights your taste buds. In this chapter, we present a variety of delicious low-carb dinner recipes that are designed to keep you feeling full and satisfied while supporting your dietary goals. From hearty main courses to flavorful side dishes, these recipes are sure to become favorites in your household.

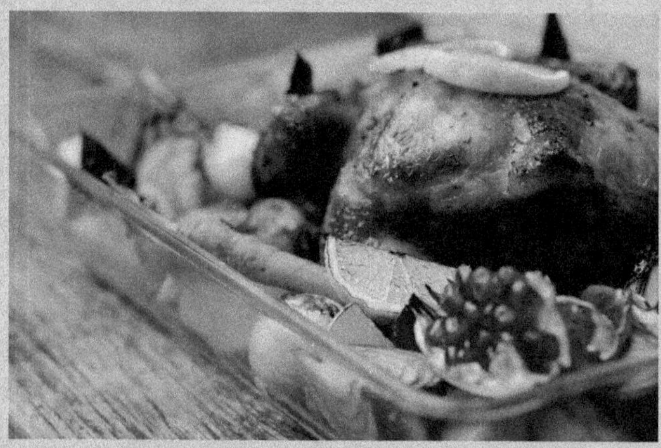

Baked Lemon Herb Salmon with Asparagus

This baked lemon herb salmon is a simple yet elegant dish that pairs perfectly with roasted asparagus. It's rich in omega-3 fatty acids and full of fresh, zesty flavors.

Ingredients:

- 4 salmon fillets
- 2 tablespoons olive oil
- 2 tablespoons lemon juice
- 2 garlic cloves, minced
- 1 teaspoon dried oregano
- 1 teaspoon dried thyme
- Salt and pepper to taste
- 1 bunch asparagus, trimmed
- **Lemon slices and fresh parsley for garnish**

Instructions:

Preheat your oven to 400°F (200°C).

In a small bowl, whisk together the olive oil, lemon juice, garlic, oregano, thyme, salt, and pepper.

Arrange the salmon fillets onto a parchment paper-lined baking sheet.

Put the asparagus in a circle around the salmon.

Over the salmon and asparagus, drizzle the lemon herb mixture.

Bake the salmon for 15 to 20 minutes, or until it is cooked through and flake readily when tested with a fork.

Before serving, garnish with lemon slices and fresh parsley.

Garlic Butter Steak Bites with Mushrooms

These garlic butter steak bites with mushrooms are a quick and delicious dinner option that's full of savory flavors. For a full supper, serve with roasted veggies on the side.

Ingredients

- 1 lb steak (such as sirloin or ribeye), cut into bite-sized pieces

- 2 tablespoons olive oil

- 4 tablespoons butter

- 3 garlic cloves, minced

- 8 ounces mushrooms, sliced

- Salt and pepper to taste

- Fresh parsley, chopped, for garnish

Instructions

- In a large skillet over medium-high heat, preheat the olive oil.

- Once the steak bites are added, grill them to the desired doneness and color. Take out and place aside from the skillet.

- Melt the butter in the same skillet over medium heat.

- When the mushrooms are soft, add the garlic and continue cooking.

- Put the steak pieces back in the skillet and toss to cover in the sauce made of garlic and butter.

- Before serving, add a dash of freshly chopped parsley and season with salt and pepper.

Zucchini Lasagna

This zucchini lasagna is a low-carb twist on the classic Italian dish. Layers of zucchini, ricotta, marinara sauce, and mozzarella make for a hearty and delicious meal.

Ingredients

- 4 medium zucchinis, thinly sliced lengthwise
- 1 lb ground beef or turkey
- 2 cups marinara sauce
- 1 cup ricotta cheese
- 1 cup shredded mozzarella cheese
- 1/4 cup grated Parmesan cheese
- 1 egg
- 2 garlic cloves, minced
- 1 tablespoon olive oil
- 1 teaspoon dried basil
- 1 teaspoon dried oregano
- Salt and pepper to taste

Instructions:

- Preheat your oven to 375°F (190°C).

- In a large skillet over medium-high heat, preheat the olive oil.

- Add the ground beef or turkey, and cook until browned. Drain any excess fat.

- Add the garlic, basil, oregano, salt, and pepper to the skillet. Stir in the marinara sauce and simmer for 10 minutes.

- Put the egg, Parmesan cheese, and ricotta cheese in a bowl.

- Using a baking dish, lightly coat the bottom with the meat sauce.

- Arrange the pieces of zucchini on top of the meat sauce.

- Spread a layer of the ricotta mixture over the zucchini.

- Repeat the layers until all ingredients are used, ending with a layer of meat sauce.

- Sprinkle the shredded mozzarella cheese on top.

- Bake for 30-35 minutes, or until the lasagna is bubbly and the cheese is golden brown.

- Let it rest for 10 minutes before serving.

Spaghetti Squash with Meatballs

A great low-carb alternative to pasta is spaghetti squash. Paired with homemade meatballs and marinara sauce, it makes for a hearty and satisfying dinner.

Ingredients

- 1 large spaghetti squash

- 1 lb ground beef or turkey

- 1/4 cup grated Parmesan cheese

- 1 egg, beaten

- 1/4 cup almond flour

- 2 garlic cloves, minced

- 1 teaspoon dried oregano

- 1 teaspoon dried basil

- Salt and pepper to taste

- 2 cups marinara sauce

- 1 tablespoon olive oil

- Fresh basil for garnish

Instructions

- Preheat your oven to 400°F (200°C).

- Scoop out the seeds after cutting the spaghetti squash in half lengthwise.

- Transfer the squash halves, cut side down, to a parchment paper-lined baking sheet.

- Bake the squash for 35 to 40 minutes, or until it's soft and shredded easily with a fork.

- Meanwhile, mix the egg, almond flour, garlic, oregano, basil, salt, pepper, and Parmesan cheese with the ground beef or turkey in a big bowl.

- Place the meatballs you formed from the mixture onto a baking sheet.

- Bake for 20 to 25 minutes, or until the meatballs are thoroughly cooked.

- In a large skillet over medium-high heat, preheat the olive oil.

- After adding the prepared meatballs and marinara sauce, simmer for ten minutes.

- Using a fork, scrape the spaghetti squash to make strands.

- Add some fresh basil as a garnish and serve the meatballs and marinara sauce over the spaghetti squash.

Alfredo chicken with broccoli

This variation of the classic comfort food, creamy chicken Alfredo with broccoli, is made with fewer carbohydrates. It has a lot of flavor and is rich and fulfilling.

Ingredients

- 2 boneless, skinless chicken breasts, sliced

- 2 cups broccoli florets

- 2 tablespoons olive oil

- 4 tablespoons butter

- 3 garlic cloves, minced

- 1 cup heavy cream

- 1 cup grated Parmesan cheese

- Salt and pepper to taste

- Fresh parsley, chopped, for garnish

Instructions

- Scoop out the seeds after cutting the spaghetti squash in half lengthwise.

- Transfer the squash halves, cut side down, to a parchment paper-lined baking sheet.

- Bake the squash for 35 to 40 minutes, or until it's soft and shredded easily with a fork.

- Meanwhile, mix the egg, almond flour, garlic, oregano, basil, salt, pepper, and Parmesan cheese with the ground beef or turkey in a big bowl.

- Place the meatballs you formed from the mixture onto a baking sheet.

- Bake for 20 to 25 minutes, or until the meatballs are thoroughly cooked.

- In a large skillet, warm the olive oil over medium heat.

- Bring the mixture to a boil after adding the heavy cream.

- Using a fork, scrape the spaghetti squash to make strands.

- Serve the meatballs and marinara sauce over the spaghetti squash, and garnish with fresh basil.

Chicken Alfredo with Broccoli

This creamy chicken Alfredo with broccoli is a low-carb version of the classic comfort food. It's full, gratifying, and dense with flavor.

Ingredients

- 2 boneless, skinless chicken breasts, sliced

- 2 cups broccoli florets

- 2 tablespoons olive oil

- 4 tablespoons butter

- 3 garlic cloves, minced

- 1 cup heavy cream

- 1 cup grated Parmesan cheese

- Salt and pepper to taste

- Fresh parsley, chopped, for garnish

Instructions

- In a large skillet, warm the olive oil over medium heat.

- Cook the chicken slices until they are thoroughly done and browned. Take out and place aside from the skillet.

- Melt the butter in the same skillet over medium heat.

- Garlic is added and cooked until aromatic.

- Bring the mixture to a boil after adding the heavy cream.

- Once the Parmesan cheese has melted and the sauce is smooth, add it and stir.

- Add pepper and salt for seasoning.

- After adding the broccoli florets, return the chicken to the skillet.

- Simmer until the broccoli is soft, about 5 to 7 minutes.

- Before serving, garnish with fresh parsley.

Bell Peppers Stuffed

A savory mixture of ground beef, cauliflower rice, and vegetables fills these stuffed bell peppers. They provide a filling and substantial supper.

Ingredients

- 4 bell peppers with the tops removed and the seeds extracted

- 1 lb ground beef or turkey

- 1 cup cauliflower rice

- 1/2 onion, diced

- 2 garlic cloves, minced

- 1 cup diced tomatoes

- One cup of shredded cheese, either mozzarella or cheddar or to taste

- 1 tablespoon olive oil

- 1 teaspoon dried oregano

- 1 teaspoon dried basil

- Salt and pepper to taste

- Fresh parsley for garnish

Instructions

- Preheat your oven to 375°F (190°C).

- In a large skillet, warm the olive oil over medium heat.

- Add the garlic, onion, and ground beef or turkey. Simmer until the onion is soft and the beef is browned.

- Add the diced tomatoes, oregano, basil, salt, and pepper, along with the cauliflower rice. Simmer for an additional five minutes.

- Take off the heat and add half of the cheese shreds.

- After packing the meat mixture inside the bell peppers, put them in a baking tray.

- Place the remaining cheese on top of the stuffed peppers.

- Bake for thirty minutes with the foil covering.

- After removing the foil, bake for a further 10 to 15 minutes, or until the cheese is bubbling and melted and the peppers are soft.

- Before serving, garnish with fresh parsley.

Thai Coconut Curry with Shrimp

This Thai coconut curry with shrimp is a flavorful and aromatic dish that's perfect for a low-carb dinner. For a full supper, serve it over cauliflower rice.

Ingredients

- 1 lb shrimp, peeled and deveined

- 1 tablespoon coconut oil

- 1 onion, diced

- 3 garlic cloves, minced

- 1 tablespoon ginger, grated

- 2 tablespoons red curry paste

- 1 can (14 oz) coconut milk

- 1 red bell pepper, sliced

- 1 zucchini, sliced

- 1 cup broccoli florets

- 1 tablespoon fish sauce

- 1 tablespoon lime juice

- Fresh cilantro for garnish

- Salt and pepper to taste

- Cauliflower rice for serving

Instructions

- In a large skillet, warm the coconut oil over medium heat.

- When aromatic, add the onion, garlic, and ginger and simmer.

- Cook for a further two minutes after stirring in the red curry paste.

- Add the broccoli, zucchini, red bell pepper, and coconut milk. Simmer for a while, or until the veggies are soft.

- When the shrimp are opaque and pink, add them and simmer.

- Add the lime juice, salt, pepper, and fish sauce and stir.

- Garnish the curry with fresh cilantro and serve it over cauliflower rice.

Stir-fried Broccoli with Beef

This flavorful stir-fry with beef and broccoli is a quick and simple dinner alternative. It's ideal for a hectic midweek dinner.

Ingredients

- 1 lb beef sirloin, thinly sliced
- 4 cups broccoli florets
- 2 tablespoons olive oil
- 3 garlic cloves, minced
- 1 tablespoon ginger, grated
- 1/4 cup soy sauce or tamari
- 1 tablespoon oyster sauce
- 1 tablespoon rice vinegar
- 1 teaspoon sesame oil
- 1 tablespoon sesame seeds for garnish
- Salt and pepper to taste

Instructions

- In a large skillet or wok, heat the olive oil over medium-high heat.

- Once added, sauté the beef until browned. Take out and place aside from the skillet.

- Add the ginger and garlic to the same skillet and sauté until fragrant.

- Stir-fry the broccoli until it becomes crisp-tender.

- Once again, add the soy sauce, oyster sauce, rice vinegar, and sesame oil to the skillet with the meat.

- Simmer for a further two to three minutes, or until thoroughly cooked and well mixed.

- Before serving, add some salt and pepper for seasoning and top with sesame seeds.

Eggplant Parmesan

This low-carb version of the traditional Italian dish is called eggplant parmesan. It's flavorful, cheesy, and rich.

Ingredients

- 2 medium eggplants, sliced into rounds

- 1 cup almond flour

- 2 eggs, beaten

- 2 cups marinara sauce

- 2 cups shredded mozzarella cheese

- 1/2 cup grated Parmesan cheese

- 1 tablespoon olive oil

- 1 teaspoon dried basil

- 1 teaspoon dried oregano

- Salt and pepper to taste

Instructions:

- In a big skillet, warm the olive oil over medium heat.
- Fry the slices of eggplant till they are golden brown on all sides. Take out and place aside from the skillet.
- Apply a thin layer of marinara sauce to a baking dish.
- Spread some eggplant slices on top of the sauce.
- Add salt, pepper, basil, oregano, mozzarella, and Parmesan cheeses.
- Continue layering until all ingredients have been used, and then top with a layer of cheese.
- Bake the cheese for 25 to 30 minutes, or until it is bubbling and melted.
- Let it rest for 10 minutes before serving.

Chicken Fajita Bowls

These chicken fajita bowls are a fun and flavorful dinner option. Serve with cauliflower rice or a bed of greens for a low-carb meal.

Ingredients

- 2 boneless, skinless chicken breasts, sliced
- 1 red bell pepper, sliced

- 1 yellow bell pepper, sliced
- 1 onion, sliced
- 2 tablespoons olive oil
- 1 tablespoon chili powder
- 1 teaspoon cumin
- 1 teaspoon paprika
- 1/2 teaspoon garlic powder
- 1/2 teaspoon onion powder
- Salt and pepper to taste
- 1 avocado, sliced
- 1/4 cup salsa
- Fresh cilantro for garnish
- Cauliflower rice or greens for serving

Instructions

- In a big skillet set over medium-high heat, warm the olive oil.
- Once the chicken is added, cook it through and until it is browned. Take out and place aside from the skillet.
- Add the onion and bell peppers to the same skillet and sauté until softened.
- Add the paprika, cumin, garlic powder, onion powder, chili powder, salt, and pepper to the skillet with the chicken once again. After combining, cook for an additional two to three minutes.
- Serve the chicken and vegetables over cauliflower rice or a bed of greens.

- Top with avocado slices, salsa, and fresh cilantro before serving.

These dinner recipes are designed to provide a variety of delicious and satisfying options that are low in carbohydrates and full of flavor. Whether you're in the mood for a hearty meat dish, a flavorful stir-fry, or a comforting Italian classic, these recipes have you covered. Enjoy these meals with your family and friends, knowing that you're nourishing your body with wholesome and nutritious ingredients

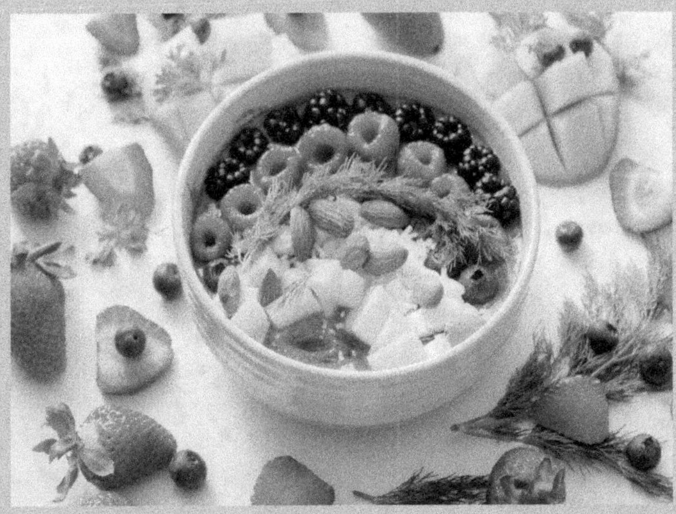

Snacks and Appetizers

Snacks and appetizers are essential parts of any diet, providing the perfect opportunity to enjoy a quick bite between meals or to entertain guests with delicious finger foods. In this chapter, we offer a selection of low-carb snacks and appetizers that are both tasty and satisfying. These recipes are designed to curb your hunger and keep your energy levels steady throughout the day.

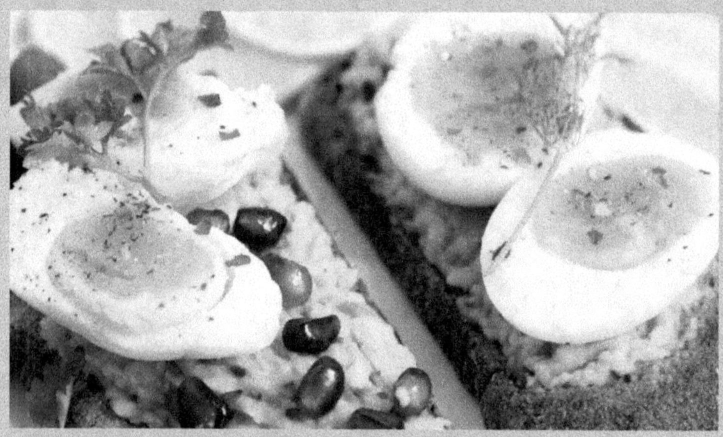

Avocado Deviled Eggs

These avocado deviled eggs are a creamy, flavorful twist on the classic recipe. These are great as a quick snack or for gatherings.

Ingredients

- 6 hard-boiled eggs, peeled
- 1 ripe avocado

- 1 tablespoon lime juice
- 1 tablespoon mayonnaise
- 1 teaspoon Dijon mustard
- Salt and pepper to taste
- Paprika for garnish
- Fresh cilantro for garnish

Instructions

- Hard-boiled eggs should be cut in half lengthwise to extract the yolks.
- Mash the avocado and egg yolks together in a bowl until they are smooth.
- Add the mayonnaise, Dijon mustard, lime juice, salt, and pepper and stir.
- In the egg whites, spoon the avocado mixture.
- Garnish with paprika and fresh cilantro before serving.

Cheese Crisps

Cheese crisps are a simple, crunchy snack that's perfect for satisfying your craving for something salty and crispy.

Ingredients

- One cup of shredded cheddar cheese (or any other hard cheese)
- Optional: spices such as garlic powder, paprika, or Italian seasoning

Instructions

- Preheat your oven to 400°F (200°C).
- Line a baking sheet with parchment paper.
- Place small mounds of shredded cheese on the parchment paper, leaving space between each mound.
- Using the back of a spoon, gently press each mound flat.
- Sprinkle with optional spices if desired.
- Bake for five to seven minutes, or until the cheese is browned and melted.
- Let the cheese crisps cool on the baking sheet before removing and serving.

Cucumber Hummus Bites

These cucumber hummus bites are a refreshing and healthy snack that's easy to prepare and perfect for any occasion.

Ingredients

- 1 cucumber, sliced into rounds
- 1 cup hummus (store-bought or homemade)
- Cherry tomatoes, halved, for garnish
- Fresh parsley or cilantro for garnish

Instructions

- Place the cucumber slices on a serving platter.

- Spoon a dollop of hummus onto each cucumber slice.
- Top with a cherry tomato half.
- Before serving, garnish with cilantro or fresh parsley.

Stuffed Mini Bell Peppers

Stuffed mini bell peppers are a colorful and tasty appetizer that's perfect for parties or as a healthy snack.

Ingredients

- 12 mini bell peppers, halved and seeded
- 1 cup cream cheese, softened
- 1/2 cup shredded cheddar cheese
- 1/4 cup chopped green onions
- 1/4 teaspoon garlic powder
- Salt and pepper to taste

Instructions

- In a bowl, combine the cream cheese, cheddar cheese, green onions, garlic powder, salt, and pepper.
- Spoon the cheese mixture into the mini bell pepper halves.
- Arrange the stuffed peppers on a serving platter and serve immediately.
-

Guacamole with Veggie Sticks

Guacamole is a classic dip that's full of healthy fats and flavor. Pair it with veggie sticks for a satisfying low-carb snack.

Ingredients

- 3 ripe avocados, peeled and pitted
- 1 lime, juiced
- 1/2 cup diced red onion
- 1/4 cup chopped fresh cilantro
- 1 jalapeño, seeded and finely chopped
- 2 garlic cloves, minced
- Salt and pepper to taste
- Veggie sticks (carrot, celery, cucumber, bell pepper) for serving

Instructions

- Mash the avocados and lime juice together in a bowl.
- Stir in the red onion, cilantro, jalapeño, and garlic.
- Season with salt and pepper to taste.
- Serve the guacamole with veggie sticks.

Prosciutto-Wrapped Asparagus

Prosciutto-wrapped asparagus is a simple yet elegant appetizer that's perfect for any occasion.

Ingredients

- 12 asparagus spears, trimmed
- 6 slices prosciutto, halved lengthwise

- 1 tablespoon olive oil
- Salt and pepper to taste

Instructions

- Preheat your oven to 400°F (200°C).
- Wrap each asparagus spear with a strip of prosciutto.
- Arrange the wrapped asparagus on a parchment paper-lined baking sheet.
- Add a drizzle of olive oil and season with pepper and salt.
- Bake for 10-12 minutes, or until the asparagus is tender and the prosciutto is crispy. Serve immediately.

Caprese Skewers

Caprese skewers are a fresh and tasty appetizer that's easy to assemble and perfect for any gathering.

Ingredients

- Cherry tomatoes
- Fresh mozzarella balls (bocconcini)
- Fresh basil leaves
- Balsamic glaze
- Salt and pepper to taste
- Skewers or toothpicks

Instructions

- Thread a cherry tomato, a mozzarella ball, and a basil leaf onto each skewer or toothpick.

- Arrange the skewers on a serving platter.
- Before serving, sprinkle with salt and pepper and drizzle with balsamic glaze.

Spicy Buffalo Cauliflower Bites

These spicy buffalo cauliflower bites are a flavorful and healthy alternative to traditional buffalo wings.

Ingredients

- 1 head cauliflower, cut into florets
- 2 tablespoons olive oil
- 1/2 cup buffalo sauce
- 1/4 cup blue cheese dressing (optional) for serving
- Fresh celery sticks for serving

Instructions

- Preheat your oven to 425°F (220°C).
- In a large bowl, toss the cauliflower florets with olive oil and buffalo sauce.
- Arrange the cauliflower evenly on a parchment paper-lined baking pan.
- Arrange the cauliflower evenly on a parchment paper-lined baking pan.
- Bake the cauliflower for 20 to 25 minutes, or until it's crispy and soft.
- Accompany with celery sticks and blue cheese dressing.

Deviled Ham Roll-Ups

Deviled ham roll-ups are a savory and satisfying snack that's perfect for any occasion.

Ingredients

- 8 slices deli ham
- 4 ounces cream cheese, softened
- 2 tablespoons Dijon mustard
- 1 tablespoon chopped fresh chives
- Salt and pepper to taste

Instructions

- In a bowl, combine the cream cheese, Dijon mustard, chives, salt, and pepper.
- On each ham slice, apply a small amount of the cream cheese mixture.
- Roll up the ham slices and secure with toothpicks if needed.
- Serve immediately or refrigerate until ready to serve.

These snacks and appetizers are designed to provide you with a variety of delicious and satisfying options that are low in carbohydrates. Whether you're looking for a quick bite between meals or a crowd-pleasing appetizer for your next gathering, these recipes have you covered. Enjoy these tasty treats while staying on track with your dietary goals

Sweet Treats and Desserts

Who says you have to give up sweets to maintain a low-carb lifestyle? In this chapter, we present a variety of delicious and indulgent desserts that are low in carbohydrates but high in flavor. From rich chocolate treats to refreshing fruity delights, these recipes will satisfy your sweet tooth without derailing your dietary goals.

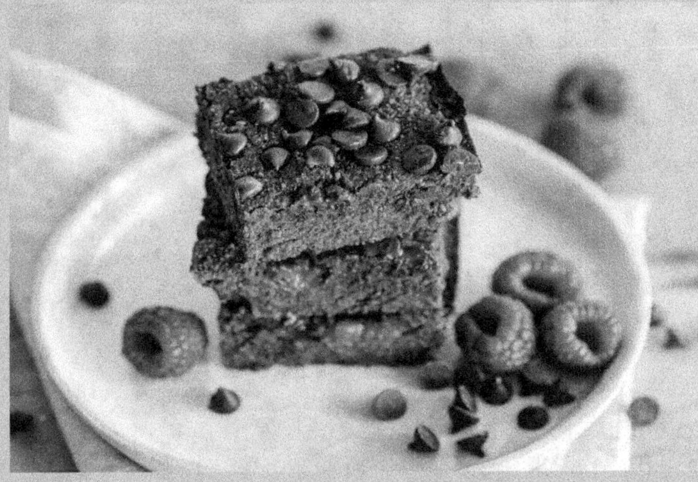

1. Keto Chocolate Brownies

Rich and fudgy, these keto chocolate brownies are really gratifying. For anyone who enjoys chocolate, these are the ideal treat.

Ingredients

- 1/2 cup butter
- 1/2 cup erythritol (or your preferred low-carb sweetener)
- 2 large eggs
- 1 teaspoon vanilla extract
- 1/4 cup almond flour
- 1/4 cup cocoa powder
- 1/2 teaspoon baking powder
- 1/4 teaspoon salt
- 1/2 cup sugar-free chocolate chips

Instructions

- Preheat your oven to 350°F (175°C).
- In a large microwave-safe bowl, melt the butter.
- Stir in the erythritol until well combined.
- Whisk in the vanilla essence and eggs until well combined.
- Mix the almond flour, baking powder, cocoa powder, and salt in a different basin.
- Mixing until thoroughly blended, gradually add the dry ingredients to the wet components.
- Fold in the sugar-free chocolate chips.
- Fill an 8 × 8-inch baking pan with batter after greasing it.
- When a toothpick put into the center comes out clean, bake for 20 to 25 minutes.
- Cool the brownies completely before slicing and serving.

2. Lemon Coconut Bars

These lemon coconut bars are a refreshing and zesty dessert that's perfect for summer or any time you crave something light and sweet.

Ingredients

- 1 cup almond flour
- 1/4 cup coconut flour
- 1/4 cup powdered erythritol
- 1/2 cup butter, melted
- 1/4 teaspoon salt
- 3 large eggs
- 1/2 cup fresh lemon juice
- 1/4 cup powdered erythritol (for the filling)
- 1/4 cup unsweetened shredded coconut
- 1 tablespoon lemon zest

Instructions

- Preheat your oven to 350°F (175°C).
- In a bowl, combine the almond flour, coconut flour, powdered erythritol, melted butter, and salt.
- Grease an 8 × 8-inch baking pan and press the mixture into the bottom of the pan.
- Bake for ten to twelve minutes, or until the crust is browned and golden.
- In a separate bowl, whisk together the eggs, lemon juice, powdered erythritol, shredded coconut, and lemon zest.

- Pour the filling over the pre-baked crust.
- Bake for an additional 20-25 minutes, or until the filling is set and golden.
- When cutting the bars into squares and serving, let them to cool fully.

3. Vanilla Chia Pudding

This vanilla chia pudding is a creamy and nutritious dessert that's easy to prepare and perfect for meal prep.

Ingredients

- 1/4 cup chia seeds
- 1 cup unsweetened almond milk
- 1/4 cup heavy cream
- 2 tablespoons powdered erythritol
- 1 teaspoon vanilla extract
- Fresh berries for topping

Instructions

- In a bowl, whisk together the chia seeds, almond milk, heavy cream, powdered erythritol, and vanilla extract.
- To avoid clumping, whisk the mixture once more after letting it settle for five minutes.
- Cover and refrigerate for at least 2 hours, or overnight, until the pudding is thick and creamy.
- Serve topped with fresh berries.

4. Chocolate Avocado Mousse

This chocolate avocado mousse is a rich and creamy dessert that's full of healthy fats and antioxidants.

Ingredients

- 2 ripe avocados
- 1/4 cup unsweetened cocoa powder
- 1/4 cup powdered erythritol
- 1/4 cup unsweetened almond milk
- 1 teaspoon vanilla extract
- A pinch of salt
- Fresh raspberries for garnish

Instructions

- Process the avocados in a food processor until smooth.
- Add the cocoa powder, powdered erythritol, almond milk, vanilla extract, and salt.
- Process the mixture until it becomes creamy and smooth.
- Spoon the mousse into serving bowls and refrigerate for at least 30 minutes before serving.
- Garnish with fresh raspberries.

5. Berry Cheesecake Bites

These berry cheesecake bites are a delightful and portable dessert that's perfect for parties or a quick snack.

Ingredients

- 1 cup almond flour
- 1/4 cup melted butter
- 2 tablespoons powdered erythritol
- 8 ounces cream cheese, softened
- 1/4 cup powdered erythritol (for the filling)
- 1 teaspoon vanilla extract
- 1/2 cup fresh mixed berries (blueberries, raspberries, strawberries)

Instructions

- Preheat your oven to 350°F (175°C).
- In a bowl, combine the almond flour, melted butter, and powdered erythritol.
- Press the mixture into the bottom of a mini muffin tin lined with paper liners.
- Roast the crust for 8 to 10 minutes, or until it turns golden brown.
- In a separate bowl, beat the cream cheese, powdered erythritol, and vanilla extract until smooth.
- Over the baked crusts, spoon the cream cheese mixture.
- Top each cheesecake bite with a few fresh berries.

- Before serving, place in the refrigerator for at least one hour.

6. Coconut Macaroons

These coconut macaroons are a sweet and chewy treat that's easy to make and perfect for satisfying your sweet tooth.

Ingredients

- 3 cups unsweetened shredded coconut
- 1/2 cup powdered erythritol
- 1/4 cup almond flour
- 4 large egg whites
- 1 teaspoon vanilla extract
- A pinch of salt

Instructions

- Preheat your oven to 325°F (165°C).
- In a large bowl, combine the shredded coconut, powdered erythritol, and almond flour.
- Whisk the egg whites until foamy in another basin.
- Stir the egg whites and vanilla extract into the coconut mixture until well combined.
- Drop tablespoon-sized mounds of the mixture onto a baking sheet lined with parchment paper.
- Bake the macaroons for 15 to 20 minutes, or until they turn golden brown.

- Let the macaroons cool completely before serving.

7. Peanut Butter Chocolate Fat Bombs

These peanut butter chocolate fat bombs are a rich and satisfying treat that's perfect for a quick energy boost.

Ingredients

- 1/2 cup natural peanut butter
- 1/4 cup coconut oil
- 2 tablespoons unsweetened cocoa powder
- 2 tablespoons powdered erythritol
- 1 teaspoon vanilla extract

Instructions

- In a microwave-safe bowl, combine the peanut butter and coconut oil.
- Microwave for 30 seconds, or until melted.
- Stir in the cocoa powder, powdered erythritol, and vanilla extract until smooth.
- Transfer the blend into ice cube trays or silicone molds.
- Freeze until solid, or for at least one hour.
- Store the fat bombs in the freezer and enjoy them as needed.

These sweet treats and desserts are designed to provide you with a variety of delicious and satisfying options that are low in carbohydrates. Whether you're in the mood for something rich and chocolate or light and fruity, these recipes have you covered. Enjoy these desserts knowing that you're indulging in treats that support your low-carb lifestyle.

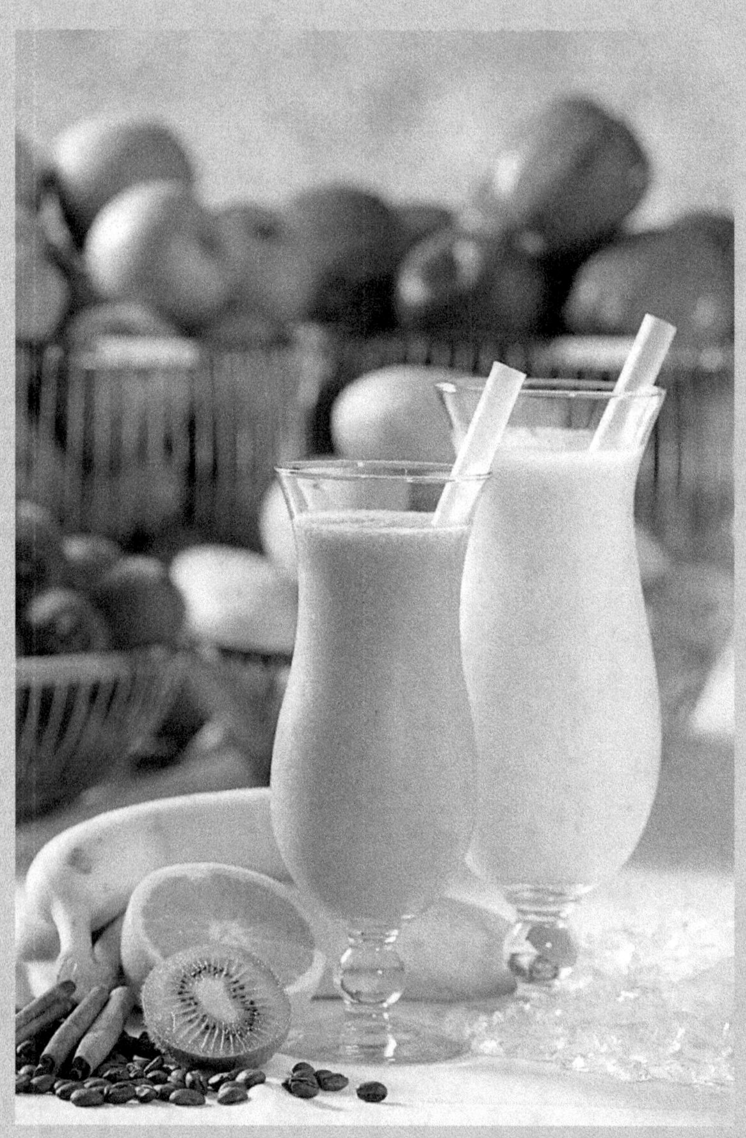

Beverages and Smoothies

Staying hydrated and enjoying delicious beverages is an important part of any diet. In this chapter, we present a selection of low-carb beverages and smoothies that are refreshing, flavorful, and satisfying. Whether you're looking for a morning pick-me-up, a post-workout smoothie, or a relaxing drink to unwind with, these recipes have you covered.

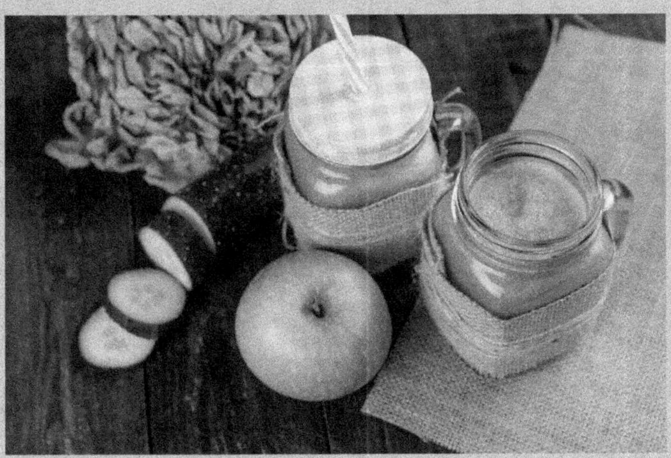

Green Detox Smoothie

This green detox smoothie is packed with nutrients and perfect for starting your day on a healthy note.

Ingredients

- 1 cup spinach
- 1/2 avocado
- 1/2 cucumber, peeled and chopped

- 1/2 green apple, cored and chopped
- 1 tablespoon chia seeds
- 1 cup unsweetened almond milk
- 1 tablespoon fresh lemon juice
- A few ice cubes

Instructions

- Place all ingredients in a blender.
- Blend until smooth.
- Pour into a glass and enjoy immediately.

Berry Protein Smoothie

This berry protein smoothie is a delicious and filling option for a post-workout snack or meal replacement.

Ingredients

- 1/2 cup mixed berries (strawberries, blueberries, raspberries)
- 1 scoop vanilla protein powder
- 1 cup unsweetened almond milk
- 1 tablespoon almond butter
- 1 tablespoon chia seeds
- A few ice cubes

Instructions

- Place all ingredients in a blender.
- Blend until smooth.
- Pour into a glass and enjoy immediately.

Iced Matcha Latte

An iced matcha latte is a refreshing and energizing drink that's perfect for a mid-afternoon boost.

Ingredients

- 1 teaspoon matcha powder
- 1 tablespoon hot water
- 1 cup unsweetened almond milk
- 1 teaspoon powdered erythritol (optional)
- Ice cubes

Instructions

- In a small bowl, whisk the matcha powder and hot water until smooth.
- Fill a glass with ice cubes.
- Pour the almond milk over the ice.
- Add the matcha mixture and stir to combine.
- Sweeten with powdered erythritol if desired.

Lemon Ginger Detox Water

This lemon ginger detox water is a refreshing and hydrating drink that's perfect for any time of day.

Ingredients

- 1 lemon, sliced
- 1-inch piece of fresh ginger, sliced
- 4 cups water
- Fresh mint leaves (optional)
- Ice cubes

Instructions

- In a large pitcher, combine the lemon slices, ginger slices, and water.
- Add fresh mint leaves if desired.
- Let the mixture sit in the refrigerator for at least 1 hour before serving.
- Serve over ice.

Coconut Matcha Smoothie

This coconut matcha smoothie is a creamy and energizing drink that's perfect for a morning boost.

Ingredients

- 1 teaspoon matcha powder
- 1/2 cup unsweetened coconut milk
- 1/2 cup unsweetened almond milk
- 1 tablespoon chia seeds
- 1 tablespoon powdered erythritol (optional)

- A few ice cubes

Instructions

- Place all ingredients in a blender.
- Blend until smooth.
- Pour into a glass and enjoy immediately.

Chocolate Peanut Butter Smoothie

This chocolate peanut butter smoothie is a rich and satisfying drink that's perfect for a post-workout snack or meal replacement.

Ingredients

- 1 scoop of chocolate protein powder
- 1 tablespoon natural peanut butter
- 1 cup unsweetened almond milk
- 1 tablespoon cocoa powder
- 1 tablespoon chia seeds
- A few ice cubes

Instructions

- Place all ingredients in a blender.
- Blend until smooth.
- Pour into a glass and enjoy immediately.

Turmeric Golden Milk

Turmeric golden milk is a warm and soothing beverage that's perfect for winding down in the evening.

Ingredients

- 1 cup unsweetened almond milk
- 1/2 teaspoon ground turmeric
- 1/4 teaspoon ground cinnamon
- 1/4 teaspoon ground ginger
- 1 teaspoon coconut oil
- 1 teaspoon powdered erythritol (optional)
- A pinch of black pepper

Instructions

- In a small saucepan, combine the almond milk, turmeric, cinnamon, ginger, coconut oil, and black pepper.
- Heat over medium heat until warm, stirring frequently.
- Remove from heat and sweeten with powdered erythritol if desired.
- Pour into a mug and enjoy.

Refreshing Cucumber Mint Water

This cucumber mint water is a light and refreshing drink that's perfect for staying hydrated throughout the day.

Ingredients

- 1/2 cucumber, sliced
- A handful of fresh mint leaves
- 4 cups water
- Ice cubes

Instructions

- In a large pitcher, combine the cucumber slices, mint leaves, and water.
- Let the mixture sit in the refrigerator for at least 1 hour before serving.
- Serve over ice.

Creamy Avocado Smoothie

This creamy avocado smoothie is a rich and satisfying drink that's perfect for breakfast or a snack.

Ingredients

- 1 ripe avocado
- 1 cup unsweetened almond milk
- 1 tablespoon chia seeds
- 1 teaspoon vanilla extract
- 1 tablespoon powdered erythritol (optional)
- A few ice cubes

Instructions

- Place all ingredients in a blender.
- Blend until smooth.
- Pour into a glass and enjoy immediately.

Strawberry Lemonade

This strawberry lemonade is a refreshing and tangy drink that's perfect for a hot summer day.

Ingredients

- 1/2 cup fresh strawberries, hulled and sliced
- 1/4 cup fresh lemon juice

- 2 cups water
- 1-2 tablespoons powdered erythritol (to taste)
- Ice cubes

Instructions

- In a blender, combine the strawberries, lemon juice, water, and powdered erythritol.
- Blend until smooth.
- Strain the mixture through a fine mesh sieve to remove any seeds.
- Serve over ice.

Vanilla Almond Milk Shake

This vanilla almond milkshake is a creamy and delicious drink that's perfect for satisfying your sweet tooth.

Ingredients

- 1 cup unsweetened almond milk
- 1 scoop vanilla protein powder
- 1 teaspoon vanilla extract
- 1 tablespoon chia seeds
- A few ice cubes

Instructions:

- Place all ingredients in a blender.
- Blend until smooth.
- Pour into a glass and enjoy immediately.

Spiced Chai Tea

This spiced chai tea is a warm and aromatic beverage that's perfect for a cozy evening.

Ingredients:

- 2 cups water
- 2 black tea bags
- 1 cinnamon stick
- 4 whole cloves
- 4 whole cardamom pods
- 1/2 teaspoon ground ginger
- 1/2 teaspoon ground cinnamon
- 1 cup unsweetened almond milk
- 1-2 tablespoons powdered erythritol (to taste)

Instructions

- In a saucepan, bring the water to a boil.
- Add the tea bags, cinnamon sticks, cloves, cardamom pods, ground ginger, and ground cinnamon.
- Reduce the heat and let simmer for 5-10 minutes.
- Remove the tea bags and strain the mixture to remove the spices.

- Return the tea to the saucepan and add the almond milk.
- Heat until warm, then sweeten with powdered erythritol to taste.
- Pour into mugs and enjoy.

These beverages and smoothies are designed to provide you with a variety of delicious and satisfying options that are low in carbohydrates. Whether you're in the mood for a refreshing drink, a creamy smoothie, or a cozy hot beverage, these recipes have you covered. Enjoy these drinks as part of your low-carb lifestyle, and stay hydrated and nourished throughout the day.

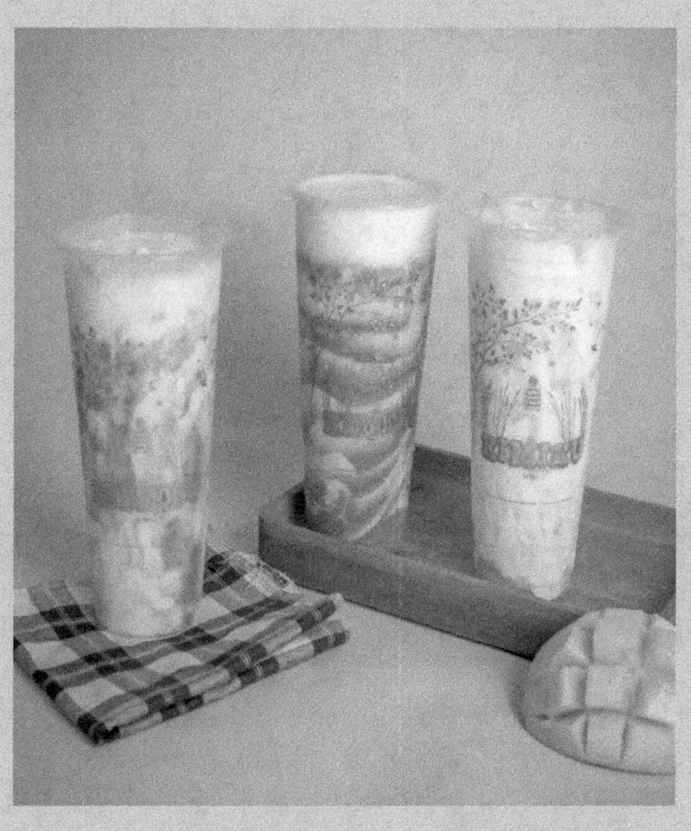

Low-Carb Sides

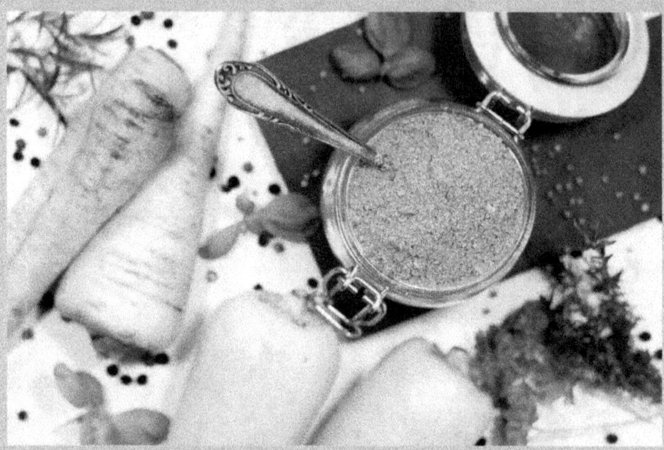

An ideal side dish would make a meal complete. This chapter offers a selection of side dishes that are low in carbohydrates and go well with any main entrée. These dishes, which range from salads and veggies to breads and other grains, are meant to enhance the taste, texture, and nutrients of your food.

Rice Made with Cauliflower

A flexible and low-carb substitute for regular rice is cauliflower rice.

Ingredients:

- 1 large head of cauliflower
- 2 tablespoons olive oil
- 1 small onion, finely chopped
- 2 cloves garlic, minced

- Salt and pepper
- Fresh parsley, chopped (for garnish)

Instructions

- Remove the cauliflower's leaves and core, then chop it into florets.
- Using a food processor, pulse the cauliflower until it looks like rice grains.
- Heat the olive oil in a big skillet over medium heat.
- Add the onion and garlic and sauté until fragrant and tender.
- Cook the cauliflower rice in the skillet for 5-7 minutes, turning regularly, until cooked.
- Season with salt and pepper to taste.
- Garnish with fresh parsley before serving.

Zucchini Noodles

Zucchini noodles, or "zoodles," are a fantastic low-carb substitute for pasta.

Ingredients:

- 2 large zucchinis
- 2 tablespoons olive oil
- 1 clove garlic, minced
- Salt and pepper
- Parmesan cheese, grated (optional)

Instructions

- Slice the zucchini into strands that resemble noodles using a spiralizer.
- In a large skillet, preheat the olive oil over medium heat.
- Garlic is added and sautéed until aromatic.
- Cook the zucchini noodles for two to three minutes, or until they are somewhat soft.
- Season to taste with salt and pepper.
- Before serving, sprinkle some grated Parmesan cheese on top if you like.

Garlic Mashed Cauliflower

Garlic mashed cauliflower is a creamy and flavorful low-carb alternative to mashed potatoes.

Ingredients:

- 1 large head of cauliflower, cut into florets
- 3 cloves garlic, peeled
- 1/4 cup unsweetened almond milk
- 2 tablespoons butter
- Salt and pepper
- Fresh chives, chopped (for garnish)

Instructions

- In a large pot, bring water to a boil and add the cauliflower florets and garlic cloves.

- Simmer the cauliflower for ten to fifteen minutes, or until it is soft.

- Drain the cauliflower and garlic and transfer to a food processor.

- Add the almond milk and butter, and blend until smooth and creamy.

- Season with salt and pepper to taste.

- Garnish with fresh chives before serving.

Spinach and Feta Stuffed Mushrooms

These spinach and feta stuffed mushrooms are a tasty and elegant side dish.

Ingredients

- 12 large mushrooms, stems removed
- 2 tablespoons olive oil
- 2 cloves garlic, minced
- 2 cups fresh spinach, chopped
- 1/2 cup feta cheese, crumbled
- 1/4 cup grated Parmesan cheese
- Salt and pepper

Instructions

- Reheat your oven to 375°F (190°C).

- In a skillet, preheat the olive oil over medium heat.

- When the spinach has wilted, add the garlic and continue to sauté.

- Remove from heat and stir in the feta cheese, Parmesan cheese, salt, and pepper.

- Stuff the mushroom caps with the spinach mixture.

- Place the filled mushrooms onto an ovenproof tray.

- Bake for 15 to 20 minutes, or until the filling is golden brown and the mushrooms are soft.

- Serve warm.

Cabbage Steaks

Cabbage steaks are a simple yet flavorful side dish that's perfect for any meal.

Ingredients:

- One large head of cabbage is cut into steaks that are one inch thick.

- 2 tablespoons olive oil

- Salt and pepper

- Garlic powder

- Fresh parsley, chopped (for garnish)

Instructions

- Preheat your oven to 400°F (200°C).

- Place the cabbage steaks in an arrangement on a parchment paper-lined baking sheet.

- Brush each steak with olive oil and season with salt, pepper, and garlic powder.

- Roast for 25-30 minutes, until the edges are crispy and golden.

- Garnish with fresh parsley before serving.

Creamed Spinach

Creamed spinach is a rich and delicious side dish that's low in carbs.

Ingredients

- 2 tablespoons butter

- 1 small onion, finely chopped

- 2 cloves garlic, minced

- 1 pound fresh spinach, chopped

- 1/2 cup heavy cream

- 1/4 cup grated Parmesan cheese

- Salt and pepper

- Fresh nutmeg, grated (optional)

Instructions

- Heat a large skillet over medium heat to melt the butter.

- Add the garlic and onion, and cook until aromatic and tender.

- Add the spinach and cook until wilted.

- Stir in the heavy cream and Parmesan cheese, and cook until the mixture is thickened and creamy.

- Add salt, pepper, and, if preferred, a small teaspoon of freshly grated nutmeg for seasoning.

- Serve warm.

Broccoli Cheese Casserole

This broccoli cheese casserole is a comforting and cheesy side dish that's perfect for any meal.

Ingredients

- 4 cups broccoli florets

- 2 tablespoons butter

- 1 small onion, finely chopped

- 2 cloves garlic, minced

- 1 cup heavy cream

- 1 cup shredded cheddar cheese

- 1/4 cup grated Parmesan cheese

- Salt and pepper

Instructions

- Preheat your oven to 350°F (175°C).

- Broccoli florets should be blanched or steamed until just soft.

- Heat a large skillet over medium heat to melt the butter.

- Add the garlic and onion, and cook until aromatic and tender.

- Cook, stirring, until the heavy cream thickens slightly.

- Remove from heat and stir in the cheddar cheese until melted and smooth.

- Season with salt and pepper to taste.

- In a baking dish, combine the broccoli florets and cheese sauce.

- Sprinkle with grated Parmesan cheese.

- Bake for 20 to 25 minutes or until bubbling and brown on top.

- Serve warm.

Ratatouille

Ratatouille is a flavorful and colorful vegetable medley that's perfect as a side dish.

Ingredients

- 1 eggplant, diced

- 1 zucchini, diced

- 1 bell pepper, diced

- 1 onion, diced

- 2 cloves garlic, minced

- 2 tablespoons olive oil

- 1 can (14.5 ounces) diced tomatoes

- 1 teaspoon dried thyme

- 1 teaspoon dried basil

- Salt and pepper

- Fresh basil, chopped (for garnish)

Instructions

- In a large skillet, preheat the olive oil over medium heat.

- Add the eggplant, zucchini, bell pepper, onion, and garlic.

- Sauté until the vegetables are tender.

- Stir in the diced tomatoes, dried thyme, dried basil, salt, and pepper.

- Simmer for 10-15 minutes, until the flavors are well combined and the sauce has thickened.

- Garnish with fresh basil before serving.

Cauliflower Mac and Cheese

Cauliflower mac and cheese is a creamy and cheesy side dish that's perfect for satisfying comfort food cravings.

Ingredients

- 1 large head of cauliflower, cut into florets

- 2 tablespoons butter

- 1/2 cup heavy cream

- 1 cup shredded cheddar cheese

- 1/4 cup grated Parmesan cheese

- Salt and pepper

- Paprika (for garnish)

Instructions

- Preheat your oven to 375°F (190°C).

- Steam or blanch the cauliflower florets until just tender.

- Heat a large skillet over medium heat to melt the butter.

- Cook, stirring, until the heavy cream thickens slightly.

- Remove from heat and stir in the cheddar cheese until melted and smooth.

- Season with salt and pepper to taste.

- In a baking dish, combine the cauliflower florets and cheese sauce.

- Sprinkle with grated Parmesan cheese and paprika.

- Bake for 20 to 25 minutes or until bubbling and brown on top.

- Serve warm.

Garlic Green Beans

Garlic green beans are a simple and delicious side dish that's quick to prepare.

Ingredients

- 1 pound green beans, trimmed
- 2 tablespoons olive oil
- 3 cloves garlic, minced
- Salt and pepper
- Lemon zest (for garnish)

Instructions

- In a large pot of boiling water, blanch the green beans for 2-3 minutes, until just tender.
- Empty and move to a bowl of ice water to cool.
- In a skillet, preheat the olive oil over medium heat.
- Add the garlic and onion, and cook until aromatic and tender.
- Add the green beans and cook for 2-3 minutes, until heated through.
- Season with salt and pepper to taste.
- Garnish with lemon zest before serving.

These low-carb side dishes will add variety, flavor, and nutrition to your meals, ensuring that you can enjoy a balanced and satisfying diet without compromising on taste.

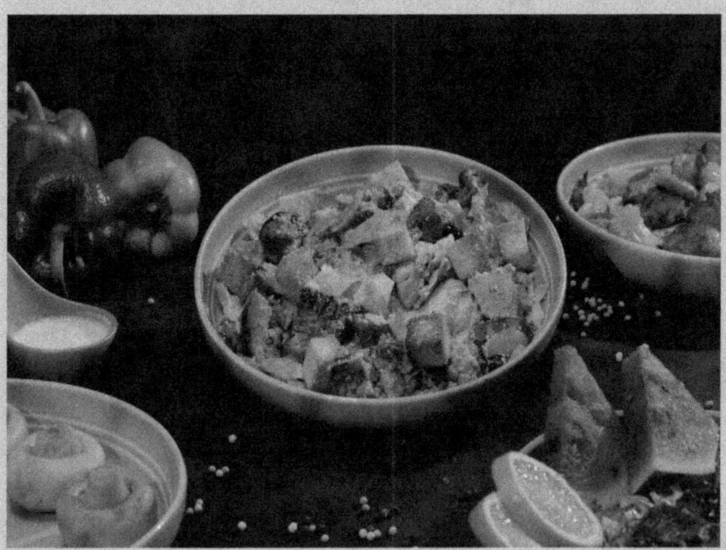

Sauces, Dressings, and Dips

The right sauce, dressing, or dip can elevate a dish from good to extraordinary. In this chapter, we provide a selection of low-carb recipes that will enhance your meals with bold flavors and rich textures. These recipes are easy to make and perfect for adding that extra something special to your salads, meats, vegetables, and snacks.

Classic Basil Pesto

Basil pesto is a versatile sauce that pairs wonderfully with everything from zoodles to grilled meats.

Ingredients

- 2 cups fresh basil leaves
- 1/2 cup grated Parmesan cheese
- 1/2 cup olive oil
- 1/3 cup pine nuts
- 3 cloves garlic, minced
- Salt and pepper to taste

Instructions

- In a food processor, combine the basil, Parmesan cheese, pine nuts, and garlic.
- Pulse until the ingredients are finely chopped.
- Olive oil should be added gradually while the machine is operating until the mixture is smooth and emulsified.
- Season with salt and pepper to taste.

- For up to a week, keep in the refrigerator in an airtight container.

Creamy Ranch Dressing

This creamy ranch dressing is perfect for salads, dips, or as a topping for grilled meats.

Ingredients

- 1 cup mayonnaise
- 1/2 cup sour cream
- 1/2 cup buttermilk
- 1 teaspoon dried dill
- 1 teaspoon dried parsley
- 1 teaspoon dried chives
- 1/2 teaspoon garlic powder
- 1/2 teaspoon onion powder
- 1/4 teaspoon salt
- 1/4 teaspoon black pepper

Instructions

- In a bowl, whisk together the mayonnaise, sour cream, and buttermilk until smooth.
- Stir in the dried dill, parsley, chives, garlic powder, onion powder, salt, and pepper.
- Cover and chill to let the flavors combine for at least 30 minutes.
- Serve chilled.

Avocado Lime Crema

This avocado lime crema is a creamy and tangy dip that's perfect for tacos, salads, or as a dip for vegetables.

Ingredients

- 2 ripe avocados
- 1/2 cup sour cream
- 1/4 cup lime juice
- 2 cloves garlic, minced
- Salt and pepper to taste
- Fresh cilantro, chopped (for garnish)

Instructions

- In a blender or food processor, combine the avocados, sour cream, lime juice, and garlic.
- Blend until smooth and creamy.
- Season with salt and pepper to taste.
- Garnish with fresh cilantro before serving.
- Store in an airtight jar in the refrigerator for up to 3 days.

Spicy Peanut Sauce

This spicy peanut sauce is perfect for dipping, drizzling over salads, or as a sauce for stir-fries.

Ingredients

- 1/2 cup natural peanut butter
- Two tablespoons of soy sauce (gluten-free: tamari)
- 1 tablespoon lime juice
- 1 tablespoon rice vinegar
- 1 tablespoon sesame oil
- 2 cloves garlic, minced
- 1 teaspoon grated ginger
- 1-2 teaspoons Sriracha (to taste)
- Water (to thin, if necessary)

Instructions

- In a bowl, whisk together the peanut butter, soy sauce, lime juice, rice vinegar, sesame oil, garlic, ginger, and Sriracha until smooth.
- Add water a tablespoon at a time to the sauce if it's too thick until you get the right consistency.
- Serve right away or keep chilled for up to a week in an airtight container.

Garlic Aioli

Garlic aioli is a rich and flavorful sauce that pairs perfectly with grilled meats, vegetables, or as a sandwich spread.

Ingredients

- 1 cup mayonnaise
- 3 cloves garlic, minced
- 1 tablespoon lemon juice
- 1 teaspoon Dijon mustard
- Salt and pepper to taste

Instructions

- In a bowl, whisk together the mayonnaise, garlic, lemon juice, and Dijon mustard until well combined.
- Season with salt and pepper to taste.
- Cover and chill to let the flavors combine for at least 30 minutes.
- Serve chilled.

Tzatziki Sauce

Tzatziki sauce is a refreshing and creamy Greek sauce made with yogurt, cucumber, and garlic.

Ingredients

- 1 cup Greek yogurt
- 1/2 cucumber, grated, and excess water squeezed out
- 2 cloves garlic, minced
- 1 tablespoon lemon juice
- 1 tablespoon olive oil
- 1 tablespoon fresh dill, chopped
- Salt and pepper to taste

Instructions

- In a bowl, combine the Greek yogurt, grated cucumber, garlic, lemon juice, olive oil, and fresh dill.
- Stir until well combined.
- Season with salt and pepper to taste.
- Cover and chill to let the flavors combine for at least 30 minutes.
- Serve chilled.

Smoky Chipotle Sauce

This smoky chipotle sauce adds a spicy kick to burgers, sandwiches, and grilled meats.

Ingredients

- 1 cup mayonnaise
- Two tablespoons of finely chopped chipotle chiles in adobo sauce
- 1 tablespoon lime juice
- 1 teaspoon smoked paprika
- Salt and pepper to taste

Instructions

- In a bowl, whisk together the mayonnaise, chipotle peppers, lime juice, and smoked paprika until smooth.
- Season with salt and pepper to taste.
- Cover and chill to let the flavors combine for at least 30 minutes.
- Serve chilled.

Lemon Tahini Dressing

Lemon tahini dressing is a creamy and tangy dressing that's perfect for salads or as a dip for vegetables.

Ingredients

- 1/4 cup tahini
- 1/4 cup lemon juice
- 2 tablespoons olive oil
- 2 cloves garlic, minced
- 1 tablespoon honey or a low-carb sweetener
- Salt and pepper to taste
- Water (to thin, if necessary)

Instructions

- In a bowl, whisk together the tahini, lemon juice, olive oil, garlic, and honey until smooth.
- If the dressing is too thick, add water a tablespoon at a time until you reach your desired consistency.
- Season with salt and pepper to taste.
- Serve right away or keep chilled for up to a week in an airtight container.

Caesar Dressing

Caesar dressing is a classic, creamy dressing perfect for salads or as a dip.

Ingredients

- 1/2 cup mayonnaise
- 1/4 cup grated Parmesan cheese
- 2 tablespoons lemon juice
- 2 tablespoons olive oil
- 2 cloves garlic, minced
- 1 teaspoon Dijon mustard
- 1 teaspoon Worcestershire sauce
- Salt and pepper to taste

Instructions

- In a bowl, whisk together the mayonnaise, Parmesan cheese, lemon juice, olive oil, garlic, Dijon mustard, and Worcestershire sauce until smooth.
- Season with salt and pepper to taste.
- Cover and chill to let the flavors combine for at least 30 minutes.
- Serve chilled.

Having a variety of sauces, dressings, and dips at your disposal can transform your meals, making them more exciting and flavorful. These low-carb recipes are designed to complement a wide range of dishes, ensuring that you can enjoy delicious and healthy meals without compromising on taste. Whether you're drizzling a salad with creamy ranch, dipping vegetables into spicy peanut sauce, or topping a grilled steak with garlic aioli, these recipes will become staples in your low-carb cooking repertoire.

Meal Plans and Shopping Lists

Embarking on a low-carb lifestyle can be made easier with a well-structured meal plan and a comprehensive shopping list. This chapter provides you with a 7-day low-carb meal plan, a detailed grocery shopping list, and tips for eating out while staying on track with your dietary goals.

7-Day Low-Carb Meal Plan

❖ **Day 1**

Breakfast: Avocado and Egg Breakfast Bowl

Lunch: Grilled Chicken Salad with Olive Oil and Lemon

Dinner: Baked Salmon with Asparagus

Snack: Cucumber Slices with Hummus

❖ **Day 2**

Breakfast: Greek Yogurt with Berries and Chia Seeds

Lunch: Tuna Salad Lettuce Wraps

Dinner: Beef Stir-Fry with Broccoli and Bell Peppers

Snack: Mixed Nuts

❖ **Day 3**

Breakfast: Almond Flour Pancakes with Sugar-Free Syrup

Lunch: Zucchini Noodles with Pesto and Cherry Tomatoes

Dinner: Roast Chicken with Brussels Sprouts

Snack: Celery Sticks with Almond Butter

❖ **Day 4**

Breakfast: Protein powder, avocado, and spinach in a smoothie

Lunch: Eggplant Parmesan

Dinner: Pork Chops with Cauliflower Mash

Snack: Cheese Slices

❖ **Day 5**

Breakfast: Chia Pudding with Coconut Milk and Strawberries

Lunch: Shrimp Salad with Avocado and Lime

Dinner: Turkey Meatballs with Zoodles

Snack: Bell Pepper Slices with Guacamole

❖ **Day 6**

Breakfast: Scrambled Eggs with Spinach and Feta

Lunch: Grilled Halloumi and Veggie Skewers

Dinner: Lamb Chops with Greek Salad

Snack: Olives and Feta Cheese

❖ **Day 7**

Breakfast: Coconut Flour Muffins

Lunch: Chicken Caesar Salad (no croutons)

Dinner: Grilled Steak with Garlic Butter and Green Beans

Snack: Dark Chocolate (85% cacao or higher)

Grocery Shopping List

Produce:

- Avocados
- Spinach
- Asparagus
- Broccoli
- Bell Peppers
- Cucumbers
- Zucchini
- Cherry Tomatoes
- Brussels Sprouts
- Eggplant
- Cauliflower
- Mixed Berries
- Strawberries
- Celery
- Bell Peppers
- Lemons
- Limes

Protein:

- Eggs
- Chicken Breast
- Salmon
- Tuna
- Beef
- Pork Chops
- Shrimp
- Turkey

- Lamb Chops
- Greek Yogurt
- Protein Powder

Pantry:

- Almond Flour
- Coconut Flour
- Chia Seeds
- Olive Oil
- Coconut Oil
- Hummus
- Almond Butter
- Peanut Butter (natural)
- Mixed Nuts
- Dark Chocolate (85% cacao or higher)
- Sugar-Free Syrup

Dairy:

- Greek Yogurt
- Feta Cheese
- Halloumi Cheese
- Cheddar Cheese
- Parmesan Cheese
- Heavy Cream
- Butter

Others:

- Pesto
- Guacamole
- Garlic

- Chia Seeds
- Canned Tomatoes
- Sugar-Free Chocolate Chips

Tips for Eating Out

1. **Plan:** Check the restaurant's menu online before you go to see what low-carb options are available.
2. **Personalize Your Purchase**: Never hesitate to request substitutions: Replace starchy sides like potatoes or rice with vegetables or a side salad.
3. **Focus on Protein and Vegetables**: Opt for meals centered around grilled meats, fish, eggs, and vegetables. Avoid breaded and fried items.
4. **Watch the Sauces and Dressings**: Ask for sauces and dressings on the side to control your intake. Choose olive oil and vinegar for salads.
5. **Skip the Bread Basket**: Politely decline the bread basket or chips served before the meal to avoid unnecessary carbs.
6. **Beverage Choices:** Stick to water, sparkling water, tea, or coffee. If you drink alcohol, choose dry wine or spirits with soda water and avoid sugary mixers.
7. **Portion Control:** Restaurant portions can be large. Consider sharing a meal, or immediately box half to take home.
8. **Dessert Alternatives**: If you crave something sweet, ask if the restaurant offers a cheese platter or a fresh berry dessert.

By following these meal plans, shopping lists, and eating-out tips, you'll be well-equipped to maintain a low-carb lifestyle with ease and confidence. Enjoy the journey to better health and delicious eating!

Maintaining Your Low-Carb Lifestyle

Embarking on a low-carb diet is a commendable step toward better health, but maintaining this lifestyle can sometimes be challenging. This chapter provides strategies to keep you motivated, tips for adjusting recipes to fit your individual needs, and an overview of the long-term health benefits of a low-carb diet.

Staying Motivated

Staying motivated is key to long-term success. Here are some strategies to help you remain committed to your low-carb lifestyle:

1. **Set Realistic Goals:** Start with achievable goals, whether it's weight loss, improved energy levels, or better blood sugar control. Reward minor accomplishments to maintain your motivation.

2. **Track Your Progress:** Keeping a food journal or using a mobile app to log your meals and progress can help you stay accountable and see how far you've come.

3. **Educate Yourself**: The more you know about the benefits of a low-carb diet and the science behind it, the more likely you are to stay committed. Read books, listen

to podcasts, and follow reputable health blogs.

4. **Find a Support System:** Join online communities or local groups where you can share your experiences, challenges, and successes. Having a network of supporters can help with accountability and encouragement.

Enjoy the Journey: Focus on the positive changes you're making rather than what you're giving up. Experiment with new recipes, try new foods and have fun with your low-carb cooking.

Adjusting Recipes to Fit Your Needs

One of the keys to maintaining a low-carb lifestyle is learning how to adjust recipes to suit your personal preferences and dietary needs. Here are some tips:

1. **Swap Carbs for Veggies:** Use vegetables like zucchini, cauliflower, and spaghetti squash as substitutes for pasta, rice, and potatoes. Spiralized zucchini makes excellent noodles, and cauliflower can be riced or mashed as a potato alternative.

2. **Use Low-Carb Flours:** Almond flour, coconut flour, and flaxseed meal are great alternatives to wheat flour in baking. They have different absorption rates, so you might need to adjust the liquid content in recipes.

3. **Choose Natural Sweeteners:** Replace sugar with low-carb sweeteners like stevia, erythritol, or monk fruit. These sweeteners provide the sweetness you crave without the added carbs.

4. **Modify Portion Sizes:** If a recipe is higher in carbs, consider reducing the portion size or pairing it with a low-carb side dish to balance out the meal.

5. **Add Healthy Fats**: Incorporate healthy fats like avocado, olive oil, coconut oil, and nuts into your meals to keep you satiated and provide essential nutrients.

6. **Experiment with Herbs and Spices:** Enhance the flavor of your dishes without adding carbs by using a variety of herbs and spices. Fresh herbs, such as parsley, cilantro, and basil, can offer a taste explosion.

Long-Term Health Benefits

Maintaining a low-carb lifestyle offers numerous long-term health benefits:

1. **Weight Management:** Low-carb diets can help you lose weight and keep it off by reducing hunger and promoting satiety. By stabilizing blood sugar levels, you're less likely to experience cravings and overeat.

2. **Improved Blood Sugar Control:** For individuals with diabetes or prediabetes, a low-carb diet can significantly improve blood sugar levels and reduce the need for medication.

3. **Enhanced Mental Clarity and Energy:** Many people report improved mental clarity and sustained energy levels on a low-carb diet. By avoiding blood sugar spikes and crashes, you can maintain consistent energy throughout the day.

4. **Better Heart Health:** Low-carb diets can improve markers of heart health, such as reducing triglycerides, increasing HDL (good) cholesterol, and lowering blood pressure.

5. **Reduced Inflammation:** A low-carb diet can reduce inflammation in the body, which is linked to various chronic diseases, including heart disease, arthritis, and certain cancers.

6. **Lower Risk of Metabolic Syndrome:** Metabolic syndrome, a cluster of conditions that increase the risk of heart disease and diabetes, can be mitigated with a low-carb diet. This includes improving cholesterol levels, blood pressure, and waist circumference.

7. **Longevity and Quality of Life:** By adopting a low-carb lifestyle, you're

investing in your long-term health. The benefits extend beyond physical health, contributing to improved mental well-being and overall quality of life.

Maintaining a low-carb lifestyle requires dedication, but the rewards are well worth the effort. By staying motivated, adjusting recipes to fit your needs, and understanding the long-term health benefits, you can enjoy a sustainable and healthy way of eating. Remember, this is not just a diet but a lifestyle change that promotes overall well-being and longevity. Cheers to your journey towards a better, healthier you!

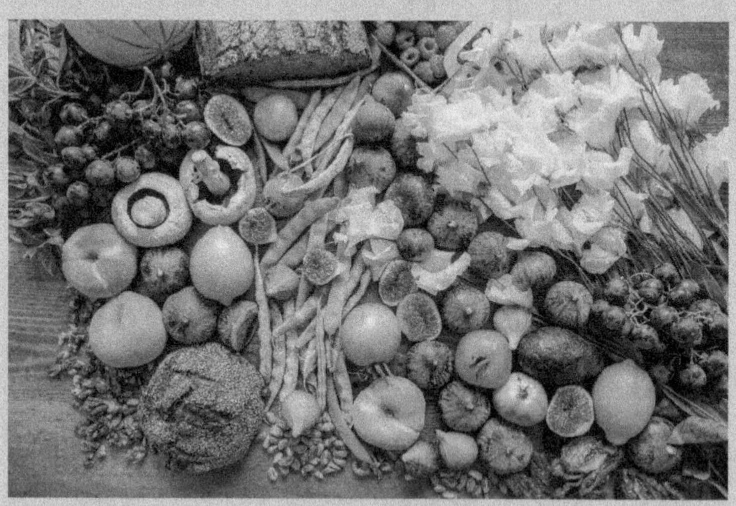

Conclusion

Low-Carbs Recipes Cookbook: Delicious and Healthy Meals for Weight Loss and Vitality. has provided you with an extensive collection of recipes, meal plans, and tips to help you thrive on a low-carb lifestyle. As you've explored the diverse and flavorful dishes, you've learned that maintaining a low-carb diet doesn't mean sacrificing taste or enjoyment.

Transitioning to a low-carb lifestyle can be a rewarding journey toward better health, improved energy levels, and a more balanced life. By incorporating the recipes and strategies in this cookbook, you're equipped to make delicious, nutritious meals that align with your dietary goals.

Remember, the key to long-term success is variety, creativity, and preparation. Don't be afraid to experiment with different ingredients, adjust recipes to your preferences, and try new dishes. The meal plans and shopping lists provided are designed to simplify your planning and ensure you always have healthy options on hand.

Whether you're cooking for yourself, your family, or entertaining guests, these recipes will make you confident in your ability to prepare satisfying low-carb meals. Enjoy the vibrant flavors, embrace the health benefits, and relish the joy of cooking and eating well.

Thank you for choosing **Low-Carbs Recipes Cookbook: Delicious and Healthy Meals for Weight Loss and Vitality** as your guide. Here's to a healthier, happier you, filled with delicious, low-carb meals every day.

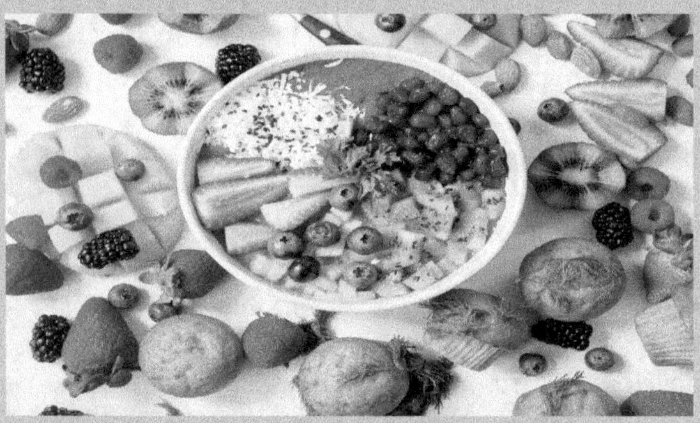